HOME-BASED CARE MINISTRY

A reflection on the challenge of HIV and AIDS to the Seventh-day Adventist Church

Judy Rose Mathers

TEACH Services, Inc.
PUBLISHING
www.TEACHServices.com • (800) 367-1844

World rights reserved. This book or any portion thereof may not be copied or reproduced in any form or manner whatever, except as provided by law, without the written permission of the publisher, except by a reviewer who may quote brief passages in a review.

The author assumes full responsibility for the accuracy of all facts and quotations as cited in this book. The opinions expressed in this book are the author's personal views and interpretations, and do not necessarily reflect those of the publisher.

This book is provided with the understanding that the publisher is not engaged in giving spiritual, legal, medical, or other professional advice. If authoritative advice is needed, the reader should seek the counsel of a competent professional.

Copyright © 2019 Judy Rose Mathers
Copyright © 2019 TEACH Services, Inc.
ISBN-13: 978-1-4796-1054-9 (Paperback)
ISBN-13: 978-1-4796-1055-6 (ePub)
Library of Congress Control Number: 2019908743

This book has been presented as a master's thesis contributing to the field of practical theology and pastoral counseling and care. The author completed her master of theology degree in clinical pastoral counseling with a specialization in HIV and AIDS ministry at the University of Stellenbosch, South Africa. The author had the privilege of successfully completing this research under the supervision and seasoned guidance of the world-renowned Professor D. J. Louw.

Published by

www.TEACHServices.com • (800) 367-1844

Dear Reader ...

This book has been written for you. The fact that you've picked it up means that you have an interest in home-based care. I am hoping to promote caring for the sick by bringing the presence of Omnipotence, Jesus Christ the Great Physician, into the homes of lonely, suffering souls Christ Himself longs to heal. My prayers are that He will bless your ministry of compassion to the ones in need to whom you have been sent to share Heaven's healing hope. You are His hands and feet to touch the world around you.

Maranatha!

"Truly I tell you, whatever you did for one of the least of these brothers and sisters of Mine, you did for Me"—Jesus (Matthew 25:40, NIV).

Drawing upon years of experience in practical theology, pastoral care and research in the field of ministry to people living with HIV and AIDS, Pastor Judy Mathers sets before us the great challenge posed by the HIV and AIDS epidemic in South Africa and outlines a way forward. The Seventh-day Adventist Church has not been spared from the ravages of this scourge! With a deep heart of love for all her fellow South Africans, she writes of the much-needed revelation of Jesus Christ in each of our communities. This book is an unfolding, in the context of home-based care ministry to people living with HIV and AIDS, of this vision cast before the church over a century ago: "Christ's method alone will give true success in reaching the people. The Saviour mingled with [people] as one who desired their good. He showed His sympathy for them, ministered to their needs, and won their confidence. Then He bade them, 'Follow Me'" (Ellen White, *Ministry of Healing*, 143). It is a heartfelt summons to the people of God to come up to the mark and love the world as Christ loved the world. You will find in these pages very practical ways to come close to your brothers and sisters in need—not only to people living with HIV and AIDS and their families affected by their illness, but to all terminally ill people and those shut-ins in our communities struggling with disease—to unload from their shoulders the weight of suffering, stigma, shame, and hopelessness, and to restore their hope and God-given dignity as children of God. The author believes that Christ's healing ministries are more effective when we bring the presence of God into the sick room. May you find *Home-Based Care Ministry: A Reflection on the Challenge of HIV and AIDS to the Seventh-day Adventist Church* to be a valuable resource in your ministry of compassion to those otherwise hurting and abandoned by society!

—Pastor Arnet Mathers, Editor

I have worked in Africa for the past 40 years—first of all in direct patient care and then in health education, disease prevention and community health promotion. As I am nearing the end of my career, I am now actively involved in global health and medical education in resource-poor countries. One of the striking deficiencies in health care in Africa is the lack of qualified health professionals, especially in the rural areas of Africa. I have promoted church-based health education and church-based community health workers for the past 40 years. In fact, I wrote a book in 1989 entitled *The Church Health Educator*. Judy Mathers' book entitled Home-Based Care Ministry is exactly what I have promoted throughout Africa. The Christian church has a strong presence in sub-Saharan Africa and properly utilized, it could compliment the traditional health services in providing simple, compassionate home care to those with HIV/AIDS. This is exactly what Pastor Mathers has so capably outlined in this book. The pastor alone has far too much responsibility to take on this role. However, properly trained members of the Christian church could make a tremendous contribution to the care of those with HIV/AIDS, relieving their suffering in all dimensions.

I would recommend that the principles outlined in Pastor Mathers' book be taken to heart both by the Seventh-day Adventist church and all other denominations as well. This is indeed the work that God has commissioned the church to do.

—Barry H. Wecker, MD MPH DTM&H FAWM

Per the referenced documents in *Home-Based Care Ministry*, Seventh-day Adventist administrative entities have addressed the scourge of HIV/AIDS. Provision is in place organizationally to do everything possible to address the situation. However, the question remains: is anyone actually doing anything about it? This book needs to be on the must-read list of every conference administrator, as well as every local congregational leader. The value of this book is in the review Judy Mathers does of the situation existing in South Africa, the country with the worst HIV/AIDS situation on the globe. Imagine: 1,000 people dying every day from HIV/AIDS, and possibly another 1,000 every day becoming infected. When you've read it and set it down, the questions you will ask yourself need to be asked.

—Dr. John Glass, Pastor for Pastoral Care
at Pioneer Memorial Church,
on the campus of Andrews University.

Dedication

The completion of this book is in no small part due to the dedication of—and is thus a tribute to—the life of my loving, late mother, Elizabeth Sophia Maria Bomester. Mom has been an icon of a virtuous woman and a stalwart in the household of faith. She always believed in me, encouraged me, and prayed for me. Mom sacrificed much to ensure a quality education for me from the time I was young. She looked forward with much anticipation to the day of my master's graduation, but sadly, she was diagnosed with breast cancer in early 2008. She suffered bravely, even when a second cancer of the lung, namely Superior Vena Cava Syndrome, robbed her of all vitality. She was a woman of faith and, like a soldier of the Cross, patiently carried her illness with courage because she believed in the resurrection. Her death on 17 April 2011 was our greatest loss; but, like Mom, I, too, will continue to live for and look forward to Christ's coming!

Table of Contents

Abstract . . . . *xv*
Acknowledgements . . . . *xviii*
Acronyms . . . . *xx*
Seventh-day Adventist Terminology and Idioms . . . . *xxii*
Abbreviations for E. G. White books . . . . *xxiii*
List of Figures . . . . *xxiv*

CHAPTER ONE
Introduction 25
1.1   Setting the Context of the Research: HIV and AIDS
in South Africa 25
1.2   Possible Challenges That Accompany an HIV and AIDS
Epidemic. 33
1.3   Home-Based Care as Supplement to Hospital Care 37
1.4   Stigma and Discrimination 42
1.5   The Role of the Seventh-day Adventist Church
in the Context of HIV and AIDS 47
1.6   Reason for Choosing This Topic 55
1.7   Problem Statement 56
1.8   Basic Research Questions 58
1.9   Basic Assumptions and Presuppositions 58
1.10 Objectives of This Research 60
1.11 Theoretical Framework. 61
1.12 Methodology 62

1.13	Scope and Limitations 63
1.14	Structure and Outline 63
1.15	Conclusion. 65

CHAPTER TWO
Introduction to the Seventh-day Adventist Church: Structure and Current Policies of the Church on HIV and AIDS 66

- 2.1 History of the Seventh-day Adventist Church in South Africa 66
- 2.2 Background 66
- 2.3 Origin of the Seventh-day Adventists in South Africa 69
  - 2.3.1 Men and Movements in the 1800s 69
  - 2.3.2 Pieter Johannes Daniel Wessels 69
  - 2.3.3 Pieter Wessels Decided to Keep the Seventh-day Sabbath 70
  - 2.3.4 George Van Druten Accepts the Seventh-day Sabbath 70
  - 2.3.5 George Van Druten and William Hunt 71
  - 2.3.6 The First Missionaries Arrive in South Africa in July 1887 72
  - 2.3.7 Organization of the Seventh-day Adventist Church in South Africa 72
  - 2.3.8 The Cape became the Headquarters of the SDA Church in South Africa. 73
- 2.4 Important Pillars in the Seventh-day Adventist Faith 73
  - 2.4.1 Education and Institutions of Learning 73
  - 2.4.2 Printing and Publishing 74
  - 2.4.3 Sanitariums and Medical Facilities 75
  - 2.4.4 The Seventh-day Adventist Church and Mission Endeavors 75
- 2.5 The Seventh-day Adventist Church Organization 76
  - 2.5.1 The Hierarchical Structure of the Seventh-day Adventist Church Organization 76

	2.5.2	The Seventh-day Adventist Church Organization as at 2004. 76
2.6	Main Areas of Work of the Worldwide SDA Church and Institutions by 2004 78	
	2.6.1	Education 78
	2.6.2	Health 78
	2.6.3	Humanitarian Work. 78
	2.6.4	Publishing Work. 78
	2.6.5	Missionary Work 79
2.7	Other Services of the Seventh-day Adventist Church 79	
2.8	The Seventh-day Adventist Church in South Africa as at 2004 80	
	2.8.1	Education 80
	2.8.2	Hospitals and Healthcare Facilities 80
	2.8.3	Humanitarian Works 80
	2.8.4	Printing and Publishing. 80
	2.8.5	Voice of Prophecy Bible Correspondence School . . . 81
2.9	The Seventh-day Adventist Doctrine on Health 81	
2.10	Adventist Healthcare Ministries and Home-Based Care—"Mi-Yittan!" 84	
2.11	Method: Jesus Christ's Method Alone Will Give True Success. 86	
2.12	The Seventh-day Adventist Church: Current Policy on HIV and AIDS. 88	
	2.12.1	General Conference of Seventh-day Adventists' Official Statement on HIV and AIDS. 88
	2.12.2	Reference Documents 91
	2.12.3	Advances Have Been Made Along Several Lines. . . . 91
	2.12.4	Official Statement of the Worldwide SDA Church on HIV and AIDS 92
	2.12.5	An Appeal as Put Forth by the General Conference 95
	2.12.6	Conclusions on the General Conference Policy on HIV and AIDS. 96

2.13	The SAU (Southern Africa Union) of SDA Working Policy on HIV/AIDS		96
	2.13.1	Name and Territory of the Association	96
	2.13.2	The Mission of the HIV and AIDS Ministries of the Southern Africa Union	97
	2.13.3	The Vision of the SAU	97
	2.13.4	The Purpose and Position Statement of the SAU of Seventh-day Adventists	97
2.14	The SAU-AAPLHA Constitution		98
	2.14.1	Name and Territory of the Association:	98
	2.14.2	Mission Statement of SAU-AAPLHA	99
	2.14.3	Vision of SAU-AAPLHA	99
	2.14.4	Aims and Objectives of SAU-AAPLHA	99
2.15	The Adventist-AIDS International Ministry (AAIM)		100
	2.15.1	The AAIM Identity Statement	100
	2.15.2	The AAIM Mission	100
	2.15.3	The AAIM Vision	101
2.16	Ellen G. White and the Care of Orphans		101
2.17	The Seventh-day Adventist Church and Health Ministries		104
2.18	Findings in Chapter Two		104

CHAPTER THREE

The HIV and AIDS Epidemic as Challenge to Other Ecclesiologies: Towards an Eclectic Contextual Home-Based Care in the SDA Church 107

3.1	HIV and AIDS: A Social Malady in South African Society	108
3.2	Five Imperative Questions Forcing Us to Come to the Party of Stakeholders of HIV and AIDS: From a Hierarchical and Clerical Structure to a Grassroots Ecclesiology	109
3.3	The JL Zwane Memorial Church, Gugulethu, Cape Town, Responds to HIV and AIDS	116

		3.3.1	The JL Zwane Mission Statement 119
		3.3.2	The JL Zwane Aims. 119
		3.3.3	The JL Zwane Home-Based Care Program. 120

3.4   An Afro-Christian Ministry to People Living with HIV
and AIDS in South Africa 121
        3.4.1   Contextual Aspects in the Afro-Christian
Approach 123
        3.4.2   The Afro-Christian Approach, Ubuntu,
and Patriarchy. 124

3.5   The Catholic Church in Rural South Africa
and HIV and AIDS. 126
        3.5.1   The Church and AIDS in South Africa
Thirty Years After the Discovery of HIV 126
               3.5.1.1   The Catholic Church Responds
to Pertinent Questions 127
               3.5.1.2   Catholic Action and Responses to the
HIV and AIDS Epidemic 130
               3.5.1.3   Challenges the Catholic Church Faces . . . 130
               3.5.1.4   The Catholic Appeal in the Face of the
HIV and AIDS Epidemic 131

3.6   Findings. 131

CHAPTER FOUR

The Seventh-day Adventist Church Within the Context of the HIV and AIDS Epidemic: Towards a Home-Based Care Model and Community-Focused Ecclesiology. 136

4.1   Pastoral Care and Healthcare Ministries to PLWHA 136
4.2   Pastoral Ministry and Care in a Multicultural
Context: South Africa 138
4.3   Important Considerations in an African Spirituality. 142
4.4   The Scripture and Theological Background
for Theory Formation. 144

	4.4.1	The Scripture and Pastoral Care as Home-Based Care. 144
		4.4.1.1 Agape Love at the Heart of Pastoral Care 145
		4.4.1.2 The Good Samaritan: Pastoral Care as Love for Neighbor 146
		4.4.1.3 Salt and Light Metaphors: Pastoral Care as Salt and Light 148
		4.4.1.4 Pastoral Care as "Immanuel, God with Us" 150
4.5	Background for Theory Formation Continued: The Spirit of Prophecy—Ellen G. White and a Ministry of Compassion 151	
4.6	Pastoral Care as "Comfort of God"—PAV Psalm 23. 158	
4.7	Louw's Theological Reframing of Power: *Cura Vitae*: Power Tools in Pastoral Care as a Way Forward in Theory Formation in Contextual Home-Based Care to PLWHA in South Africa 163	
4.8	Training Caregivers to Help PLWHA in Coping with Illness as an Art 167	
4.9	God-images in Spiritual Healing. 169	
	4.9.1 Four Metaphors: God-images 171	
4.10	Spirituality and Spiritual Healing 173	
4.11	An Existential Approach: *Cura Vitae*—Life Dimensions of Healing. 175	
	4.11.1 Existential Dimensions of Life 175	
	4.11.2 Schematic Summary: *Cura Vitae*—Life Dimensions of Healing 177	
	4.11.3 Promissio Therapy 179	
4.12	Home-Based Care Programs in the Seventh-day Adventist Church: An Answer to the Challenge of HIV and AIDS in South Africa 180	
4.13	Research Findings 185	

4.14	Recommendations	187
4.15	Further Study	191
4.16	Conclusion	191

Appendices

Appendix 1: Organizational Structure of the Seventh-day Adventist Church 194

    SAU Pastoral Statistics Report 194
        Pastoral Statistics 195
        Internship 197
        Ordinations 197
        Withdrawal of Credentials and Resignations 198
        Ministerial Employees' Meetings and Conventions 198
        Training Programs and Resources 198
        Pakia, Shepherdesses, And Retired Pastors. 199
        Appreciation 201
    Ratio of Pastors to Churches and Members 202
        Cape Conference 202
        Kwazulu Natall-Free State Conference 202
        Lesotho Conference 203
        Namibia Conference 203
        Northern Conference (Formerly Transvaal Conference) . . . 203
        Swaziland Conference 204
        Trans-Orange Conference 204

Appendix 2: Departments in the Seventh-day Adventist Church for Ministry 205

        Children's Ministries 205
        Communication 205
        Education 205
        Family Ministries 206
        Health Ministries 207
        Public Affairs and Religious Liberty 207

    Publishing Ministries 207
    Sabbath School 208
    Personal Ministries 208
    Stewardship Ministries 208
    Women's Ministries. 208
    Youth Ministries 209

Bibliography. *211*

Abstract

This book primarily concerns itself with HIV and AIDS as a challenge to the Seventh-day Adventist Church in South Africa and is reflection on home-based care to people living with HIV and AIDS (PLWHA). On 01 December 2014, International AIDS Day, *eNCA* (eNews Channel Africa) released the staggering statistics which revealed that South Africa has the most serious HIV and AIDS epidemic in the world, with 6 million South African PLWHA in an estimated population of 54 million, whereas only 2.7 million of these PLWHA were receiving proper treatment and care. The Department of Health (DOH) reported that there were 1,000 new infections and more than 1,000 AIDS-related deaths daily in 2014. Despite South Africa being the leading nation in HIV and AIDS research, the country has the highest rate of infections and disease-related deaths—less than half of the South African PLWHA are receiving treatment.

These staggering reports of the sobering reality of the South African situation on the HIV and AIDS epidemic ought to be seen as the wakeup call to faith communities in South Africa, including the Seventh-day Adventist Church. Church leaders of all denominations are faced with the same challenge of their members living with HIV and AIDS, and the Seventh-day Adventist Church is not spared. The Seventh-day Adventist Church must therefore become a visible, active stakeholder in making a difference in the campaign against HIV and AIDS. The primary aim of this book is to examine how the Seventh-day Adventist Church in South Africa can help bring relief to the burden of illness and suffering, poverty, helplessness, and shame, and empower vulnerable PLWHA and their family members through the formulation of contextual Home-Based Care programs.

The core focus of this book is on existing policies in the Seventh-day Adventist Church and it questions the theological and ecclesiological implications for being "church" in poor communities where care facilities and health facilities are lacking. It is in this regard that the option of a Home-Based Care model surfaces. Study is given on how the Seventh-day Adventist Church in South Africa should restructure its current policies in order to shift from a clerical model to a more community-oriented model of pastoral care to PLWHA. The author challenges the Seventh-day Adventist Church to live up to the light it has been given regarding pastoral care, healthcare, and other ministries to spiritually and physically sick people, by preparing and training their lay members as volunteers in doing Home-Based Care to PLWHA in South Africa. Despite the continued advances in the fields of science, medicine, and associated professional health care services, the challenges of human diseases in epidemic proportions, more specifically HIV and AIDS, still present us with a need to care for persons, families, and communities afflicted with illnesses. An urgent need exists to respond to the quest for meaning in human suffering and the restoration of human dignity, before God, in our approaches to ministry and therapy, reaching across the cultural divides.

This book extensively expounds on the mandate of the Scriptures as the primary and pivotal calling of the church to engage in medical missionary work to PLWHA. Pastoral care strategies in a multicultural society are adequately discussed as essential for contextual ministries to the people of South Africa. The importance of sensitivity to and education in African spirituality is addressed and various theories of Professor Daniël Louw,[1] author of *A Pastoral Hermeneutics of Care and Encounter, A Theological Design for Basic Theory, Anthropology, Method, and Therapy*, and *Cura Vitae*, are presented as power tools in pastoral care and should be of great help to the Seventh-day Adventist Church in South Africa in the

---

[1] https://1ref.us/rv (accessed 5/6/2019).

formulation of a successful Home-Based Care ministry as a new ecclesial direction to an HIV and AIDS ministry have been cited.

The culture of the gospel is one that sees the former barriers of racial divides and African cultural differences or indifferences as opportunities for spiritual healing, growth, and transcendence in setting us free, and moving the Seventh-day Adventist Church in South Africa towards truly being and becoming *koinonia* to PLWHA: a place where God's grace lives. The church of God on earth in every aspect and manner of being is the place where *Agape love*, unconditional acceptance, healing and forgiveness, spiritual encounter, reconciliation, worship of God the Creator, and eschatological hope of the advent of Christ's coming bring us all, sinners and saints alike, into the priesthood of believers and into unity of community in Christ.

In Christ we are all one ... Father make us one!

Acknowledgements

My highest praise, gratitude, thanks, and honor go to God, Jehovah Jireh! Indeed, the Lord has carried me through. The journey has been great, though extremely tough at times, with many a challenge and even some painful experiences, amongst which were the long illness and loss of my dear, loving mother. But God continued to prove faithful throughout the journey. Thank you, Lord Jesus, for calling me to this course of study. Surely, You have blessed me with the health and strength, the means, the courage, and endurance to complete this mammoth task.

I owe a great debt of gratitude to my children—Stafford and Olivia, Emile, Robin and Deidre, and Jody—and to my grandchildren—Jayrid, Tristan, Isabella, and Ezra. Thank you for holding my calling in high regard and believing in me. Thank you for granting me the time and space which I could dedicate to study and research. Your love, patience, prayers, sacrifices, understanding, and support in every way mean the world to me. Emile, you assumed a unique role during this time by helping me raise Jody and getting him through high school. My siblings, Arthur, Trevor, Gloria, and Wilhelmina, thank you for always being there for me. I love you all!

I wish to acknowledge Professor Daniël Louw for his guidance and the patience he has shown during my years of study at Stellenbosch University. In Prof. Louw, I have found a true counselor and pastoral leader in the academic discipline. I would also like to thank the Church of Sweden for sponsoring me on the master of theology program. Without their initial funding it would basically have been impossible for me to conduct this research study.

To the most amazing editor ever, who became my Love, Pastor Arnet Clare Mathers, Calais, Maine, USA—you truly became the wind beneath my wings! Thank you for your laborious hours of reading, editing, faithful assistance, and your love. May God reward you greatly!

Many thanks to my friends, Dr. Jakes Carnow, Ds. Lee-Ann Simon,[2] and Dr. Moira Bladergroen, who supported me and encouraged me to finish this thesis, especially when things seemed too overwhelming for me. Dr Josiah Murage, your amazing example of endurance is still an inspiration to me. Thank you for helping me to stay focused. Finally, to my extended family, a host of friends, and the members of the Seventh-day Adventist Church in South Africa and abroad for their continued prayers and support throughout my time of study—thank you.

---

[2] Official abbreviation for "Dominee," a minister in the Dutch Reformed Church in South Africa.

Acronyms

AIDS—Acquired Immunodeficiency Syndrome
AAIM—Adventist AIDS International Ministry
AAPLHA—Association of Adventist People Living with HIV and AIDS
ANC—Antenatal Care
CBO—Community-Based Organization
CBVCT—Community-Based Voluntary Counselling and Testing
CHC—Community Health Center
CHBCP—Contextual Home-Based Care Programs
CIRCLE—Circle of Concerned African Women Theologians
FBO—Faith-Based Organization
HAART—Highly Active Antiretroviral Therapy
HBC—Home-Based Care
HIV—Human Immunodeficiency Virus
HIVAN—Center for HIV/AIDS Networking
NGO—Non-Governmental Organization
PLWHA—People Living with HIV and AIDS: reference to People Living with HIV and AIDS. "PLWHA" wherever used in this paper is inclusive of all races, both within the Seventh-day Adventist Church and non-members, in all South African communities.
PMTCT—Prevention of Mother-to-Child Transmission
Ps—Pastor
SACC—South African Council of Churches
SAQA—South Africa Qualifications Authority
SDA—Seventh-day Adventist

TB—Tuberculosis
UNAIDS—The Joint United Nations Program on HIV and AIDS
VCT—Voluntary Counselling and Testing
WHO—World Health Organization

Seventh-day Adventist Terminology and Idioms

AAIM—Adventist AIDS International Ministry
ADRA—Adventist Disaster and Relief Agency
Advent Movement—The Seventh-day Adventist Church as a people
Adventurers—Department of the Church catering to 5–9-year olds
Ambassadors—Department of the Church catering to 16–19-year olds
AWM—Adventist Women's Ministries
AY—Advent Youth (20–30-year olds)
GC—General Conference World Headquarters of Seventh-day Adventists
HM—Health Ministries
Pathfinders—Department of the Church catering to 10–15-year olds
PM Ministries—Personal Ministries Department of the Church
Sanitarium—Medical facility caring for in/out-patients
SAU—Southern Africa Union
SAU-AAPLHA—SAU Association of Adventist People Living with HIV and AIDS
SDA—Seventh-day Adventist
SS—Sabbath School Department
SOP—Spirit of Prophecy
VOP—Voice of Prophecy Bible School

Abbreviations for E. G. White books

AA—*The Acts of the Apostles*
CD—*Counsels on Diet and Foods*
CH—*Counsels on Health*
DA—*The Desire of Ages*
FW—*Faith and Works*
GC—*The Great Controversy*
GW—*Gospel Workers*
Lt40-1899—Letter #40, 1899 (dated 23 February 1899)
MH—*The Ministry of Healing*
13MR—*Manuscript Releases*, vol. 13
Ms43-1901—Manuscript #43, 1901 (dated 1 April 1901)
RH—*Review and Herald/Advent Review and Sabbath Herald*
1SM—*Selected Messages*, Book 1
6T—*Testimonies for the Church*, Vol. 6

List of Figures

Figure 1	Organizational Structure of the Seventh-day Adventist Church	77
Figure 2	God-images: Symbols with Corresponding Concepts of God and Possible Effects	171
Figure 3	*Cura Vitae*: Cure of Soul as Life Dimensions	176
Figure 4	*Cura Vitae*: Christian Spiritual Care and healing as the Pastoral Response to Existential Threats	178

CHAPTER ONE

Introduction

1.1 Setting the Context of the Research: HIV and AIDS in South Africa

This chapter is aimed at giving an introduction to the book as a whole. It consists of the background to the study, the statement of the research problem, limitations of the research, objectives, methodology, basic assumptions, and presuppositions. An outline of the chapters is also provided. In this book I examine the HIV and AIDS epidemic as a challenge to the Seventh-day Adventist Church in South Africa and will reflect on contextual Home-Based Care and pastoral care to PLWHA. Wherever the term "PLWHA," is used throughout this book it refers to all people living with HIV and AIDS and is inclusive of all races, both within the Seventh-day Adventist Church and non-members in all South African communities.

The truth about the conversation on the topic of HIV and AIDS is that this infectious disease is a human condition, which to date has been categorized as an incurable infectious disease—and is therefore an ongoing dialogue for the stakeholders of HIV and AIDS management. HIV and AIDS has reached epidemic proportions in many countries around the world and in South Africa this is no exception. While it is true that HIV and AIDS affect some communities more adversely than others, this is a topic which we cannot ignore. Because HIV and AIDS is a widespread reality for the South African society, every citizen should live in awareness of the far-reaching effects of the disease and regard themselves as stakeholders of a campaign against HIV infection.

On 01 December 2014, International AIDS Day, *eNCA* (eNews Channel Africa) released these staggering statistics that reveal South Africa has the most serious HIV and AIDS epidemic in the world:[3]

1. At July 2014, Statistics South Africa (Stats SA) estimated the population of South Africa to be fifty-four million with an HIV prevalence of 17.9 percent.
2. At the time more than six million South Africans were living with HIV (the biggest epidemic in the world) and only 2.7 million of those PLWHA were receiving treatment, and that largely because of the work that the Treatment Action Campaign (TAC) has done.
3. The Department of Health reported that there were 1,000 new infections and more than 1,000 AIDS-related deaths daily in 2014.
4. Southern Africa has the most serious HIV and AIDS epidemic in the world. A little over thirty years ago, it was virtually unheard of in the region, but now, it is regarded as the "epicenter" of the global HIV epidemic.
5. Despite South Africa being the leading nation in HIV and AIDS research, the country has the highest rate of infections and disease-related deaths—less than half of South African PLWHA are receiving treatment.

In July 2015, Stats SA reported the South African population to be 54.9 million. As was the case in 2014, the Black African population remained in the majority at 44.23 million, or 80 percent of the total population, with Whites estimated at 4.53 million, Coloureds[4] at 4.83 million and Indians/Asians at 1.365 million.

---

[3] https://1ref.us/rw (accessed 5/6/2019).
[4] https://1ref.us/rx (accessed 5/6/2019).

Despite being known as a global leader in HIV research,[5] South Africa still experiences problems such as a lack of HIV and AIDS knowledge and education, a low rate of condom use in monogamous relationships, early sexual debate, and HIV-related risk behavior.

According to *eNCA*, the Human Sciences Research Council (HSRC) report named a few important focal areas for change, namely:

I. Condom use and sufficient distribution,
II. An increase in knowledge of HIV,
III. Regular testing (and maintaining awareness of one's status), and
IV. The stigma and discrimination, especially when referring to PLWHA as the "other."

These are all areas that need constant work and attention in order to decrease prevalence and risk of infection.

These staggering reports of the sobering reality of the South African situation on the HIV and AIDS epidemic ought to be seen as the wake-up call to faith communities in South Africa, including the Seventh-day Adventist Church. Church leaders of all denominations are faced with the same challenge of their members living with HIV and AIDS, and the Seventh-day Adventist Church is not spared. The Seventh-day Adventist Church must therefore become a visible, active stakeholder in making a difference in the campaign against HIV and AIDS.

It has become clear that after the demise of apartheid, the church[6] in South Africa has found itself faced by the greater challenge of HIV and AIDS, which has silently entrenched itself in the socio-economic and political structures. The Joint United Nations Programme on HIV and AIDS (UNAIDS) has shown that South Africa has one of the highest

---

[5] https://1ref.us/rw (accessed 5/6/2019).
[6] Wherever the term "church" is used throughout this book, it refers to the general Christian church, that is, all Christian denominations. Whereas in instances when reference is made to the "Seventh-day Adventist Church," the name will be written out in full, or the acronym "SDA Church" will be used.

rates of HIV-AIDS worldwide.[7] According to South African History Online, March 2011, over five-and-a-half million people are already infected with the HI virus, and almost 1,000 AIDS deaths occur every day. Factors leading to this high-ceilinged growth are varied.

However, the socio-economic structures of apartheid not only created an environment conducive to the epidemic—taking into consideration the township revolts of the 1980s and the migrant labor system that coincided with the epidemic—but it also relegated the HIV and AIDS epidemic to the side-line as politics of transition took center stage. This was done in the interest of both the outgoing regime and its incoming nationalist successor.[8] The nature of the apartheid system was such that it ensured black people were denied the right to own businesses. The political struggle, especially in the 1970s and 1980s, seriously disrupted and impaired educational opportunities for blacks. Thus, many people were robbed of the opportunity to acquire skills that would enable them to be employed in the financial sector. Walshe affirms that during that period, "the overcrowding in the classrooms was not conducive to effective education since the government was also not supportive of black education."[9] He noted that differences in the occupancy of classrooms between the whites and blacks were 25:90 respectively. Most students of the class of 1976 are referred to as "the lost generation" because those who did not go into exile or join the ANC's armed wing, "*UmkhontoWesizwe*," were left with

> "It has become clear that after the demise of apartheid, the church in South Africa has found itself faced by the greater challenge of HIV and AIDS, which has silently entrenched itself in the socio-economic and political structures."

---

[7] UNAIDS/WHO (2010), 2.
[8] Iliffe (2006), 41.
[9] Walshe (1995), 68.

no education and could not be employed.[10] This added to the already high number of people who were unemployed in South Africa. Despite the emergence of the new government after 1994, the high rate of unemployment prevailed. This is because most of the Blacks were people of low income with an unemployment rate of 40%.[11] In other words, one contributing factor was that apartheid had actively impoverished most black people, a situation not easily reversed by the new incoming government, and this poverty made them susceptible to the HIV and AIDS epidemic.[12]

In addition to the above, the migratory labor system brought about the emergence of single-sex hostels, hence providing an atmosphere conducive to the spread of the HI virus. Walshe observes that one third of the African workforce were men living without their families, which further contributed to family disorganization and to men engaging in sex with multiple partners.[13] The apartheid policy of the Nationalist Government broke down the cohesiveness of the black family with its values pertaining to extended family life, which provides protection to orphans.[14] Walshe describes the brutal character of urban policy in this way:

> It is accepted government policy that Bantu are only temporarily resident in the European areas of the Republic, for as long as they offer their labour there. As soon as they

---

[10] Ibid.

[11] Census 2001.

[12] In terms of poverty, the World Bank (2009:4) defines poverty as "a multidimensional phenomenon, encompassing inability to satisfy basic needs, lack of control over resources, lack of education and skill, poor health, malnutrition, lack of shelter, poor access to water and sanitation, vulnerability to shocks, violence, crime, lack of political freedom and voice." Poverty seriously challenges the way we manage the disease because the consequences of poverty are extensive. For instance, unemployment, poor living conditions, poor healthcare facilities and lack of education all propel people to make the wrong choices in their struggle to survive. Poverty creates or breeds conditions in which, for example, women tend to engage in prostitution for survival. More specifically, poverty generally creates conditions that are conducive to the erosion of sexual morality and sexual customs that exist between men and women because of the strain that poverty creates. Therefore, it can be argued that poverty leads to an increase in unsafe sexual encounters, which are not considered risky because the most important issue on women's minds is to put food on their tables.

[13] Walshe (1995), 68.

[14] Thomas and Mabusela (1991), 121.

> become, for some reason or other, no longer fit for work or superfluous in the labour market they are expected to return to their country of origin or the territory of the national unit (Bantustan) where they fit in ethnically if they were not born or bred in the Homeland.[15]

He also notes that such apartheid policies could only be enforced by the institutionalized and recurring harassment of black people by police and other officials continued when checking that they were "lawfully" in particular areas.[16] The result of the above was prosecutions on a large scale: "Savage's calculations indicate that between 1946–1964/5 a total of 6 million were prosecuted for pass law offences."[17] And as seen above, these policies were deliberately designed to make the cities and towns as unattractive for blacks as possible. Similarly, the policies were intended to prevent the development of stable families with communities in the white areas.

Apart from the constant aggravation of pass law enforcement, Walshe affirms that black people were subjected to:

> [N]ight-curfews and other regulations, the effort to freeze the urbanized black population took other forms, including: limitation on the scope of black traders, who were, in any case confined to black townships; the phasing out of sub-economic (subsidised) housing after 1958; the abolition in 1968 of the right of urban blacks to lease property on a 30 year leasehold agreement; the requirement that 'nie-plekgebonde' (locality bound) institutions in white areas, including certain types of hospital, old age homes, and homes for the blind and deaf, must be transferred to the "homeland"; the limitation after 1959 on the expansion

---
[15] Walshe (2009), 62.
[16] Ibid.
[17] Ibid.

of secondary and technical schools for blacks in the white areas; from 1968 onwards the supply of urban housing for blacks was drastically reduced, being replaced by the construction of barrack like hostels for single migrants; and from 1958 onwards a policy directive required that township houses be allocated strictly according to ethnic group.[18]

Because of the above dysfunctional system, there was an increase in cross-border migration and many blacks were displaced from their homes. This forced them to seek refuge in other countries totally outside South Africa. This cross-border migration caused a breakup of family units and provided fertile ground for the spread of the HI virus. In fact, it should be noted that the contributions made by the apartheid regime to the disruption of family life, which only allowed women a two-weeks per annum conjugal visit to their husbands who lived in the single sex hostels, was another fertile ground for the spread of the HI virus. Clapp asserts that the above dysfunctional system also resulted in single parenthood by creating a situation where about 19% of household partners lived elsewhere far from the family due to migrant working conditions. It is said that 42% of mothers and 50% of fathers did not live in the same households as their children.[19]

Children who are brought up this way often end up in institutions or live on their own while others survive through social welfare. The result of such separation between children and their parents is poor socialization whereby children do not learn the societal norms that include family values and life skills that would protect them from falling prey to social ills. Today, many teenagers and young women live together with their boyfriends outside of wedlock, hence engaging in high-risk sexual behavior.

The above shows that the HIV and AIDS epidemic came at a bad time for the newly established South African democracy. Mamphela Ramphele notes that "it bore all the hallmarks of a spoiler of the hard-won freedom."[20]

---

[18] Ibid.
[19] Clapp et al (2011), 12.
[20] Ramphele (2008), 227.

Ramphele wondered how the young South African democracy can face the challenges posed by the HI virus. She asks:

> How can our young democracy manage the risks this pandemic posed to reconstruction and development, given its strong sexual undertones, and given that we are uncomfortable talking about sex? How could we manage the risks it presented without reinforcing the stereotypes about black people and their sexual mores?[21]

While the questions posed are varied, it is observed that the slow response in the 1990s of the South African government to the escalating wave, and particularly its failure to take advantage of pharmaceutical discounts on antiretroviral medicines in 2000s, have been roundly criticized.[22]

Des Martin provides, probably, the most inclusive articulation and critique when he says:

> South Africa is host to a burgeoning HIV epidemic of catastrophic proportions. The country has the dubious honour of having the most HIV-infected individuals in the world. The roots of the [pandemic] are complex and lie within a web that embraces poverty, lack of empowerment of women, gender violence and the legacy of the apartheid era. This has led to migrant workers, single-sex hostels and fragmentation of the normal family structures that would be protective in this epidemic. The epidemic in South Africa has further been fuelled by the inaction of both past and present governments and has spawned a society that has discriminated against and stigmatised those who suffer from the disease.[23]

---

[21] Ibid.
[22] Barnett and Whiteside (2002), 298; cf. Patel (2001), 79–90.
[23] Martin (2006), 10.

Following former President Thabo Mbeki's unprecedented denial that AIDS is caused by HIV, critics earmarked the country, internationally, as "a country in denial."[24] During his time, Mbeki supported views of discredited "dissident" scientists such as Duesburg, Resnick, and Mhlongo, who challenge the theory that AIDS is caused by a virus.[25] This was coupled with Minister of Health Manto Tshabalala Msimang's persistent proclamations that "African vegetables," such as beetroot, sweet potato, and garlic, rather than anti-retroviral treatment, are effective antidotes for improving the immune systems of PLWHA.[26] Such declarations send confusing messages to the public and point to a lack of clear direction, which impedes "the creation of an imaginative, yet workable national strategy for approaching a problem," that requires serious and urgent attention.[27]

By and large, the South African HIV and AIDS story is one that encapsulates an intriguing debate and an abject denial in the face of a fast unfolding spate of the epidemic. In fact, it is difficult to exaggerate the suffering that HIV has caused in South Africa. In view of the startling fact that one in every five adults in South Africa is said to be infected, and the rapid spread of the virus, it is becoming very difficult for many people inside and outside South Africa to imagine an effective response.[28] It is becoming more difficult to envisage an effective way to care for all the PLWHA and to curtail the epidemic.

1.2 Possible Challenges That Accompany an HIV and AIDS Epidemic

In the late 1990's, upon entering the homes of PLWHA as a pastoral volunteer, I became aware of the various challenges that accompany an HIV and AIDS epidemic, of which the increasing number of orphans is

---

[24] Whiteside and Clem (2001), 1.
[25] Van Niekerk (2001), 143.
[26] Ibid.
[27] Ibid.
[28] UNAIDS/WHO (2011), 2.

one. Van Dyk predicted that by 2010 there would be 2.2 million children orphaned by AIDS and by 2015 the number would be 3.1 million—that is 18 percent of the total number of children under the age of eighteen in South Africa.[29] The situation in South Africa as reported by UNICEF[30] is that the country is experiencing the highest burden of HIV in the world, with over 5.7 million people currently infected. It is only when caring for PLWHA in their homes that one becomes aware of the vulnerability of their children. Parents are dying and leaving behind orphaned children. Currently there are an estimated 3.7 million orphans in South Africa, about half of whom have lost one or both parents to AIDS, and 150,000 children are believed to be living in child-headed households.[31] Most of these orphans are traumatized by the illness of their parent(s) in addition to the stigma and discrimination attached to HIV and AIDS. A good Home-Based Care program would put pastoral caregivers in touch with these orphans. UNICEF presents a list of some other experiences these children have that will assist Christian churches in knowing how to care for their needs in their homes:[32]

a) **Economic hardship:** With parents unable to work and savings spent on health care, children are forced to take on the adult role of supporting the family.
b) **Having to leave school:** The pressures of having to care for parents and siblings while trying to earn an income causes them to drop out of school, even while their parents are still alive. The pressure to abandon schooling intensifies when one or both parents die.
c) **Malnutrition and illness:** Orphans and other affected children are more likely to be malnourished and sometimes they become ill. They are also less likely to receive the medical attention and healthcare they need. Poverty is the root cause of this vulnerability, but often neglect

---

[29] Van Dyk (2008), 269.
[30] 2015.
[31] https://1ref.us/ry (accessed 5/6/2019).
[32] UNICEF (2011), 2.

and discrimination by adults in whose care they have been left, are also contributing factors.
d) **Loss of inheritance:** When parents die, orphans are often cheated out of property and money that are rightfully theirs.
e) **Fear and isolation:** Dispossessed orphans are often forced out of their homes to unfamiliar and even hostile places, be they camps for the displaced or the streets.
f) **Increased abuse and risk of HIV:** Impoverished and without parents to educate and protect them, orphans and other affected children face every kind of abuse and risk, including becoming infected with HI virus themselves. Many are forced into exploitative and dangerous work, including exchanging sex for money, food, protection, or shelter.

In rural areas the most prevalent problems affecting AIDS orphans are lack of education and problems regarding transport, poverty, and unemployment. In addition, some live with the HI virus. While some orphans were born before their parents were infected with HIV, others were not lucky enough to escape it and were infected because their mothers did not have access to AZT[33] to prevent pediatric transmission or Mother to Child Transmission (MTCT). Although some orphans did not contract the HI virus because they underwent this program, most of these children head the family or they care for the dying parents with no adult support. Van Dyk argues that in circumstances where children have become caregivers to adults with HIV and AIDS, their childhood is effectively sacrificed.[34] She goes on to say that these children "grow without parental care and love" and most of them are "deprived" of their basic rights to shelter, food, health, and education.[35] And because the greatest

---

[33] AZT: Zidovudine, Retrovir is an anti-HIV drug that reduces the amount of virus in the body, slows down or prevents damage to the immune system, and reduces the risk of developing AIDS-related illnesses. Oral medication.
[34] Van Dyk (2008), 269.
[35] Ibid.

challenge faced by these children is finding sufficient food, housing, and health care, the church and the community can play a decisive role in showing love and care.

Churches in communities can help to bring relief to the burden of poverty, helplessness, and shame, and empower vulnerable family members—especially children of PLWHA—through serving meals and training programs in "finding and using resources outside of oneself [themselves], in such a way as to enable them to think and act in ways that will result in greater freedom and participation in the life of the societies of which they are a part."[36] As much as *empowering the poor* might have become a slogan around the world, in South Africa the increasing poverty as a result of the HIV and AIDS epidemic is a reality that cannot be ignored.

> *"Churches in communities can help to bring relief to the burden of poverty, helplessness, and shame, and empower vulnerable family members."*

I make use of the following basic assumptions for focusing on HIV and AIDS as an ecclesial problem which all Christian churches should address, including the Seventh-day Adventist Church. A number of needs can be addressed by Christian churches when we enter into the homes of PLWHA. Therefore, there is a need for the Seventh-day Adventist Church in South Africa, as a faith community, to take the initiative of training their members in supporting children who are fulfilling adult roles—often at the expense of their own security and development. Indeed, the Seventh-day Adventist Church can play a vital role in formulating multi-dimensional Home-Based Care programs that can, amongst other things, enable families and orphans to avoid or prevent:

a) Serious threat to education because of poverty;
b) Difficulty in obtaining food and shelter;

---

[36] Lartey (2003), 68.

c) High risk of being sexually abused by relatives and neighbours;
d) Threat of child prostitution and child labour;
e) Difficulty in getting birth registration done and in procuring healthcare and social security benefits;
f) Experiencing property grabbing by families and communities.

In addition to the above, the needs of orphans, children, and family members of PLWHA are among the multiplicity of needs of the millions of victims living with HIV and AIDS in South Africa for which the Seventh-day Adventist Church can investigate possible intervention strategies through Home-Based Care projects. These Home-Based Care projects can also help to alleviate some of the challenges associated with hospital care to PLWHA from poor communities.

1.3 Home-Based Care as Supplement to Hospital Care

Although with antiretroviral drug treatment, those living with HIV and AIDS can live a relatively "normal" life, these drugs are only accessible to a very few people compared to the number of people who need these drugs. Because of the serious shortage of hospital beds in South Africa, accommodating all the people with both AIDS-related and other diseases not related to HIV and AIDS has become a challenge—"In both the private and the public sectors South Africa is struggling with a tremendous shortage of hospital beds."[37] What this means is that something needs to be done to help those who suffer from AIDS-related diseases because many people are now dying at home. According to *The New York Times* of 19th December 2011, AIDS-related diseases cause almost half of all deaths in South Africa and 71 percent of these deaths occur among those who are between 15 and 49 years of age. Some church denominations in South Africa have even commented that there are more funerals than weddings

---

[37] 2010, *Huge shortage of hospital beds*, fin24archives, https://1ref.us/rz (accessed 5/6/2019).

in the church today.[38] There is a need, therefore, for a different care system because hospital care should be supplemented by Home-Based Care.

Going by the above figures and acknowledging that both the community and individuals are suffering because of the HIV epidemic, the Adventist AIDS International Ministry (AAIM)[39] of South Africa has unanimously agreed that the Seventh-day Adventist Church cannot sit down and see people dying at home without any help or care. Further, the Seventh-day Adventist Church has noted that many of its members are also living with HIV and AIDS and this is a challenge to the church. Hence it can no longer ignore the HIV and AIDS epidemic. The HIV and AIDS Ministries Department of the South African Union (SAU) of Seventh-day Adventists have as their Working Policy on HIV and AIDS mission statement[40] the following:

> To coordinate actions and resources to bring comfort, healing and hope to people infected and/or affected by HIV/AIDS, share a message of education and prevention to the SAU territory, and to accomplish what our Lord Jesus Christ has commissioned each of us to do.

Alongside their mission statement, the vision statement[41] of the SAU:

1. To create "Centers of Hope and Healing" through our network of churches, medical and educational institutions.
2. To mobilize our congregations through church-based support groups.
3. To bring practical solutions to those infected and affected by HIV and AIDS.
4. To apply the practical Gospel of Jesus Christ, church-by-church, person-by-person, and one-to-one.

---

[38] Johnson (2006), 6.
[39] https://1ref.us/s0 (accessed 5/6/2019).
[40] HIV/AIDS Ministries, Southern Africa Union, "Working Policy on HIV/AIDS."
[41] Ibid.

Inasmuch as AAIM has a worthy policy in place to care for AIDS sufferers around the world, the Seventh-day Adventist Church in South Africa is faced with unique challenges such as:

1. The challenge of the massive workload of district pastors which makes it impossible to reach and effectively care for PLWHA.[42] Appendix #1 is a 2015 report of the SAU Ministerial Association of the SDA in South Africa giving a clear indication of the great challenge overburdened pastors have caring adequately for their members. In Table 1 of the report the pastoral statistics show their pastor-to-member ratio as 1:554.
2. The challenge that most of the PLWHA are living in the poorest areas of the country where reaching and caring for them is most difficult. Even though the majority of the Church's membership is also there, the resources from which to draw are limited by the prevailing economic conditions of the area.
3. The challenge of a racially merged Seventh-day Adventist Church in South Africa since 2005 is that it is still seemingly focused on administrative issues in its attempts to save the church organization, leading to its failure to mobilize its members effectively in ministries to PLWHA.

Similarly to the AAIM mission and vision statement, the SAU Working Policy on HIV and AIDS[43] also defines ministries to PLWHA as a clear framework within which the Southern Africa Union will:

> Provide guidelines for the church leaders on how to relate and minister to people living with HIV in their congregations and communities, create church based support, and mobilise their congregations for a Ministry of Compassion.

---

[42] See Appendix #1: *Report of the Ministerial Association Presented to the Fifth Business Session of the SAUC*.
[43] https://1ref.us/t4 (accessed 5/6/2019).

The SAU of Seventh-day Adventists also:

- Acknowledges the seriousness of the HIV and AIDS epidemic and the potential negative impact it presents to the organization and all aspects of society.[44]
- Recognises the direct link between infection by HIV and Sexually Transmitted Infections (STI's) as well as sexual intercourse. And stipulates that this will be part of the education for all denominational employees, volunteers, students, and church members, as far as is reasonably possible. (SAU policy 3.5)
- Seeks to set forth the responsibility of both the church organization and church leaders to educate their employees, students and members regarding HIV and AIDS, including modes of transmission and means of prevention. (SAU policy 3.6)
- Seeks, within its means, to minimise the social, economic and developmental consequences of HIV and AIDS on communities, the organization, and God's people. (SAU policy 3.7)
- Is committed to providing hope, love and support to all employees, students, church members and members of the community who are diagnosed as being HIV positive, so as to assist them to continue to live a dignified and productive life for as long as possible. (SAU policy 3.8)
- Will provide counselling for employees, students and members who are affected, in an attempt to improve their overall health; approaching those infected with compassion and respect. (SAU policy 3.9)
- Is committed to providing protection and assistance to women, children, youth and vulnerable groups. (SAU policy 3.10)

Furthermore, the SAU has undertaken that "the leadership and administrative personnel of the Southern Africa Union should monitor and periodically review *their* policy. Workplace and industry standard

---

[44] Ibid.

updates on the issues encompassed in *their* policy should be identified and incorporated at regular intervals."[45]

However, in my experience and observation over a number of years of the effectiveness of the Seventh-day Adventist Church in terms of their HIV and AIDS policies converting these into interventions and programs caring for the PLWHA, it has become clear that their policies appear good but lack its implementation due to the following:

1. The contents of its policies not being communicated to their congregations and members on a grassroots level. At the end of the day these are the ones primarily responsible for taking charge of Home-Based Care programs and reaching PLWHA in churches and in the communities.
2. Some of its churches, leaders, and members are still oblivious and ignorant in regards to the seriousness of the crisis of an HIV and AIDS epidemic within the borders of South Africa.

It would appear that the above challenges which the unified Seventh-day Adventist Church in South Africa are facing are all effects of the aftermath of the merger of their conferences in South Africa; similar challenges would be experienced in other denominations countrywide where unification occurred. Much of the resources and energies of the Seventh-day Adventist Church are still spent on *saving the administrative structure of the church while millions of PLWHA in South Africa are suffering and dying, including its own members at a grassroots level.*

Besides intensifying the prevention against HIV programs, the Seventh-day Adventist Church has a mission to care for those PLWHA who are sick and dying among their members as well as their families affected by the HIV and AIDS epidemic in South Africa. I believe that intensified educational programs for its members in HIV and AIDS ministries and introducing Home-Based Care strategies are vital as a new ecclesial

---

[45] Ibid.

direction to empower and equip the church in making a more meaningful contribution to PLWHA, both in the church and in the community. This would also help the Seventh-day Adventist Church to apply and align itself with the HIV and AIDS policies held by the larger Seventh-day Adventist Church worldwide.

Alongside the challenges of orphaned children, and the need for Home-Based Care as supplementary care to hospital care for PLWHA, the issue of stigma and discrimination cannot be overlooked in a holistic addressing of pastoral care to PLWHA. These realities that accompany a ministry to PLWHA must be taught to all pastoral caregivers to ensure an effective, compassionate Home-Base Care ministry.

1.4 Stigma and Discrimination

A further serious challenge facing the Seventh-day Adventist Church in South Africa in the context of HIV and AIDS is the issue of stigma and discrimination. Of course, discrimination and stigma have always been present in the world. In a post-apartheid South Africa, the persisting issue of stigma and discrimination needs serious attention, which the Church should address. Stigma was a strong social force even in the Greek world and still is a great challenge among the people of South Africa. Page argues that:

> "Stigma" dates back to the Greek word for "tattoo-mark," which was a brand mark made with a hot iron and impressed on people to show that they were devoted to the services of the temple, or, on the opposite spectrum of behaviour, that they were criminals or runaway slaves. These marks were used somehow to expose the infamy or disgrace of people who had sinned (sic) against society and God.[46]

---
[46] Page (1984), 2.

Because many people die of AIDS-related illnesses in Africa, most PLWHA have been stigmatized. Philip sees stigma as an unhealthy attitude, which discredits the basic human integrity of the person in society due to a condition or sickness to which he or she is subjected.[47] In fact, judgmentalism and rumor-mongering have been described as classic examples of how the PLWHA are labelled as immoral people. Prof. Louw argues that, "With a society, the question as to how the person became infected by the virus, often remains unmasked, for infection as such already implies a stigma...."[48] Even the question of how the HI virus was contracted is "part and parcel of the problem of stigmatization."[49]

When HIV and AIDS emerged in South Africa in the 1980s, the media perception was that of male homosexuality playing a major role. Therefore, homosexuals were seen as responsible for the epidemic.[50] Later both PLWHA and homosexuals were lumped together and seen as one and the same thing. This means that PLWHA are likely to be labelled as gay, hence running the risk of being judged and stereotyped without confirming evidence. Prof. Louw argues that due to common assumptions, a sufferer is believed either to have behaved shamefully or to be morally at fault and therefore deserving of punishment.[51]

The judgments associated with HIV and AIDS are fueled by the paradox of the fundamental connection between life-creating sexuality and death, which has a strong effect on people. Luchetta sees a stigma "as a mark or brand of shame that has been elaborated by social scientists to refer to the social label conferred upon individuals or groups by virtue of their possession of a characteristic indicative of a deviant condition."[52] Chitando is of the opinion that stigma also follows the fault-line of gender inequality.[53] He goes on to explain that in most parts of Southern Africa,

---

[47] Philip (2006), 330.
[48] Louw (2008), 401.
[49] Louw (2006), 398.
[50] Ibid.
[51] Louw (2008), 334.
[52] Luchetta (1999), 4.
[53] Chitando (2008b), 183.

sexually transmitted infections are referred to as "women's diseases." Thus, women who are infected with the HI virus are often viewed as promiscuous and thus discriminated against. If women are open about their HIV status, they are likely to be the talk of the village or even the church community.

Hence, women or other people infected by HIV would prefer to keep it secret. Therefore, the existence of stigma hampers any efforts that are designed to stem the tide of the HIV and AIDS epidemic. The condition of deviance is said to disrupt social interaction and is even "perceived by others as repellent, ugly or upsetting."[54] In fact, the last stages of HIV infection can have a dramatic effect on the physical appearance and vitality of individuals, which may result in distress and in discrimination by others[55] Theories of HIV and AIDS-related stigma developed by social psychologists often describe two sources for individual attitudes concerning the HIV- and AIDS-related stigmas. Herek describes possible sources and functions of an HIV- and AIDS-related stigmatizing attitude.

> *"The existence of stigma hampers any efforts that are designed to stem the tide of the HIV and AIDS epidemic."*

The first source of attitude results in an "instrumental HIV and AIDS stigma," which is the attitude of the instrumental stigma grounded in the fear of HIV and AIDS as a disease, and an accompanying desire to protect oneself from it due to its infectiousness and lethality. Stigma based on fear functions as a means of protection against the disease.

The second source of stigmatizing attitude is the symbolic association between HIV and AIDS and groups identified with the virus. A "symbolic HIV and AIDS stigma" exists due to social meanings attached to HIV and AIDS. The latter "represents the use of the disease as a vehicle for expressing a variety of attitudes like negligence or ignorance." Basic to the

---

[54] Herek (2010), 110.
[55] Herek (2010), 111.

symbolic stigmas are social meanings connected to norms and values of a society.⁵⁶ According to UNAIDS:

> Stigma is linked to power and dominion throughout society as a whole. It plays a key role in producing and reproducing relations of power. Ultimately, stigma creates and is reinforced by social inequality. It has its origins deep within the structure of society as a whole, and in the norms and values that govern much of everyday life. It causes some groups to be devalued and ashamed, and others to feel that they are superior.⁵⁷

For example, long-standing ideologies of gender have resulted in women being blamed for the transmission of sexually transmitted infections or HIV. This has influenced the ways in which families and communities react to the sero-positive women. Many are blamed for the illness from which they and their husband suffer.

Chitando notes that, "Stigma discourages people living with HIV or AIDS from seeking care and support as they fear discrimination." This shows that stigma is very dangerous to people living with HIV and AIDS. It is a burden for many women, especially those who are in a culture that demeans them and where people lack understanding and openness about HIV and AIDS. This means that the church has an obligation to fight stigma and discrimination if the fight against HIV and AIDS is to be won.

When confronting the HIV and AIDS stigma, Ackermann claims that there are two categories of stigmatization. First is the "brutal" and "violent" one, while the second is understood as that which manifests with "great subtlety."⁵⁸ She affirms that both may have a distressing effect on the human being. Ackermann further states that the starting point in dealing with stigma and its effects is to become aware of its complexity;

---

⁵⁶ Herek (2010), 112.
⁵⁷ UNAIDS, https://1ref.us/s1 (accessed 5/6/2019).
⁵⁸ Ackermann (2006), 4.

understanding stigma becomes the "first line of defense."[59] For Prof. Louw, "[S]tigmatisation and labelling are synonymous with immediate isolation. HIV therefore becomes the leprosy of the twenty-first century."[60]

On an existential and social level, rejection means exclusion from community, in life and closeness to death, "which is the ultimate state of loneliness."[61] If HIV/AIDS is the leprosy of the 21st century,[62] then stigma can be understood as the stone people throw at one another—*"let the one who has never sinned throw the first stone."*[63] The aspect of attitude is intrinsic to human beings, whereas the quality of attitude is varying. Attitude finds orientation in norms and values. The pastoral challenge should therefore be to establish the norm of the will of God; as such destigmatization presumes an overhaul of a person's normative system. As we have seen above, the HIV- and AIDS-related stigma points to "pre-existing stigmata" like the racism created by apartheid, poverty, sexuality, and gender.

So far this research study has uncovered the reality, seriousness, and the rapid spread of HIV and AIDS in epidemic proportions in South Africa. Several challenges that link poverty, medical, and health care needs to HIV and AIDS as well as educational and empowerment of Seventh-day Adventists, as discussed in 1.3–1.4 above, bring us to the question of the role of the Seventh-day Adventist Church in South Africa in the spate and context of HIV and AIDS.

In retrospect, the merged Seventh-day Adventist Church in South Africa has a need to train their leaders, pastors, and members on how to address issues of increasing stigmatization that accompanied restructuring. If the Seventh-day Adventist Church claims to be the church of God on earth, then there is no place for discrimination and stigmatization as

---

[59] Ibid.
[60] Louw (2007), 401.
[61] Louw (1998), 3.
[62] Louw (2008), 60.
[63] John 8:7, NLT.

we all are one before God and all members—especially PLWHA—should know and feel that they belong to the body of Christ, which is the church.

There is a definite link between poverty, HIV, and AIDS. I have intentionally highlighted these challenges above in order to draw the attention of the Seventh-day Adventist Church to pivotal areas of concern both in the church and in the community where pastoral care, counselling, and a ministry of compassion to PLWHA are needed and long overdue. The stigmatization issue in particular could possibly raise its ugly head as the challenge of restructuring and rethinking the ecclesial framework and paradigm with the Seventh-day Adventist becomes a necessity. I see the need for the introduction of multi-dimensional Home-Based Care to PLWHA as a move in the right direction to assist pastoral staff with the problem of HIV and AIDS and the communities where they serve.

1.5 The Role of the Seventh-day Adventist Church in the Context of HIV and AIDS

The importance of the role of the churches as households of faith in the context of the HIV and AIDS epidemic in South Africa cannot be overemphasized. Both the church and the government have continually been under the spotlight with regards to their response to the epidemic. In other words, all the religious institutions have a role to play in responding to health crises by creating the individual, communal, cultural, socio-economic, and environmental conditions that can enhance and maintain the health of those living with HIV and AIDS. This means that the role of religious institutions has to be recognized in dealing with HIV and AIDS, and this is so particularly within the religious community itself. In fact, the religious institutions have enormous assets which they could mobilize in an effort to create good health conditions while facing the challenges of the HIV and AIDS epidemic.

In this book there will be an attempt to reflect on the role the Seventh-day Adventist Church in South Africa can play in addressing these and other challenges posed by the HIV and AIDS epidemic. It will be argued that the notion of the idea of the extended family system which traditionally provides support for the vulnerable and which is embedded in the African "ubuntu" culture is crucial in helping the church create programs through *"koinonia"*—the community and fellowship of believers functioning as the body of Christ on earth where ministry, communion, fellowship, joint participation, and sharing that which one has in anything, through gifted ministries, is spiritual worship expressed in daily life and experience—geared towards supporting PLWHA and ones affected.

This is because the increasing effects of the HIV and AIDS epidemic jeopardize the rights and well-being of orphans and PLWHA. As seen above, the responsibility of caring for orphans has become a major problem in South Africa because poverty and unemployment have made it difficult for families and extended families to cope with the orphans. Therefore, the ecclesiological praxis of the Seventh-day Adventist Church in South Africa, within the context of HIV and AIDS epidemic, cannot be ignored.

"If the Seventh-day Adventist Church claims to be the church of God on earth, then there is no place for discrimination and stigmatization as we all are one before God and all members—especially PLWHA—should know and feel that they belong to the body of Christ, which is the church."

The above observation was affirmed by theologians such as Prof. Louw, Ronald Nicolson, Willem Saayman, and Jacques Kriel, who in the early 1990s argued that the church (i.e., all Christian denominations in South Africa) was better positioned to respond to the epidemic given that it was, in contrast to the apartheid government, trusted by the majority and the disadvantaged population, and that it had a well-established structure in the communities—right from the grassroots.[64] However, they lamented, "The churches,

---

[64] Louw (1991; 1994); Nicolson (1995), 7; Saayman; and Kriel (1991).

who proclaim the Word, were at a loss for words in the face of HIV and AIDS pandemic."[65] It is likely, however, that not all churches lacked words in the face of HIV and AIDS epidemic. Most certainly, some found words and actions to respond to it.

Earlier, the Seventh-day Adventist church attempted to respond to the challenges posed by the HIV and AIDS epidemic. The General Conference of Seventh-day Adventists released their GC-AIDS policy in 1990[66] which was distributed to its divisions and unions worldwide,[67] but the Church in South Africa spent considerably more time on the issue of a merger of all its conferences in South Africa. In fact, many church denominations were busy reorganizing themselves to adapt to and influence the new government under former president Nelson Mandela. For instance, in July 1990, the Catholic bishops met in Pietermaritzburg to reflect on the role of the church in the new dispensation. At the same time, the Methodist Church of South Africa was busy amending her constitution, which strongly advised rejection of the government's constitution and to reject any system that would support the entrenched sin of apartheid in the referendum.[68] Before that, since the 1980s, most churches worked towards peace and promoted racial equality, human rights, and the worth of a democracy. In 1986 some of the leaders of the white Dutch Reformed Church started rejecting the official policy on race relationships here in South Africa.

In April 1990 the Anglican Archbishop of the Cape, Bishop Desmond Tutu, and the Dutch Reformed Church, made a public confession asking for forgiveness for sins committed during apartheid. In other words, all church denominations in South Africa were coming to terms with the promising sense of freedom but they took a long time to initiate programs to fight the HIV and AIDS epidemic. There has been a general failure of

---

[65] Nicolson (1995), 7.
[66] https://1ref.us/t5 (accessed 5/6/2019).
[67] See Figure 1: Organizational Structure of the Seventh-day Adventist Church, p. 77 of this book.
[68] The White Referendum 1983. Fact Sheet 16, https://1ref.us/s2 (accessed 5/6/2019).

all societal structures (governmental, communal, tribal, and ecclesial) to prevention and treatment of the HIV and AIDS epidemic. South African government policies have created major obstacles to an effective prevention and treatment program that to date have in large measure overpowered the ability of effective communal, tribal, and ecclesial response. At the same time, the societal stigma attached to PLWHA has seriously undermined the capacity for compassion, love and commitment necessary to mount effective help at any level of society.

In summary, Mathers[69] stated:

> In other words, the tribal, familial, and church norms and structures that would have strengthened the family unit and protected the populace from high risk behaviors, have been so hampered by governmental policies of apartheid, and the economic and structural legacies of those policies in post-apartheid South Africa, as to be rendered almost totally ineffective.

Thus, it has also become increasingly apparent that the solution to the HIV and AIDS epidemic is no longer simply a biomedical one, but it also involves an interrogation of the social contexts in which the epidemic thrives. In South Africa this proves to be a major challenge, especially in addressing the underlying problem of poverty and a lack of strong leadership to deal with such issues. It has also become clear that despite knowing how HIV and AIDS are transmitted, people still engage in high-risk sexual behavior. The same challenge is facing the Seventh-day Adventist Church in South Africa.

The inability of people to change their sexual behavior has forced the Seventh-day Adventist Church to adopt an HIV and AIDS campaign based on abstaining and reminding them to be faithful to one partner. The Seventh-day Adventist Church generally upholds in its teaching a

---

[69] Mathers, Arnet C. Calais, Maine (2015).

positive view of sexuality that encourages the importance of building solid and positive relationships between married couples, and therefore discourages sexual intimacy before marriage.[70] The Seventh-day Adventist Church has long advocated premarital abstinence and has limited sexual intercourse to the heterosexual marriage relationship. However, it sees the physical, social, psychological, and healthcare needs of PLWHA as very important, and advocates that its members, pastors, and leaders have a moral obligation to PLWHA, and therefore encourages its pastors, leaders, and members to treat all PLWHA with dignity, compassion, and respect. In the NGO circles, there is the ABC[71] campaign where they emphasize "**A**bstain, **B**e faithful, and use a **C**ondom." However, neither of these formulas has succeeded in curbing the rate of HIV infections in South Africa. The problem with models that adhere to the ABC theory in the context of the HIV and AIDS epidemic is that they send the message to people that the prevention of this epidemic is possible if sexual partners behave more carefully. In this way, the issue of sexual morality is seen as if it is an individual responsibility, while in a very real sense it is communal in nature.

In both campaign models the target is the individual and the model relies on individual morality and individual responsibility. This individualistic thinking comes from Western philosophy as illustrated by René Descartes, who says, "I think therefore I am" (*cognito ergo sum*)[72] and it is opposed to communal African thinking as exemplified by Mbiti.[73] The idea of oneness, the "we" and "us," is ingrained in the African, and compels a person to work and live within a community. For Mbiti, the African philosophy is, "I am, because we are; and since we are, therefore I am" or "I am related, therefore, I am" (*cognatus ergo sum* or an existential *cognatus sum, ergo sumus*, that is, "I am related, therefore, we are").[74]

---

[70] https://1ref.us/t4 (accessed 5/6/2019).
[71] https://1ref.us/s3 (accessed 5/6/2019).
[72] Russell (1991), 547
[73] Mbiti (1969), 4; cf. Berinyuu (1988), 5, and Bujo (1998), 186.
[74] Mbiti (1969), 108.

In fact, Benezet Bujo states that: "When the news spread around the world like a bush-fire that a new and incurable, deadly virus had been discovered, the age-old moral model was reviewed: i.e., AIDS must be a punishment or scourge of God against the sexual dissoluteness of our world. This scapegoat morality justly caused resentment."[75] He adds that such perceptions generated the arguments that those who got HIV were being punished for their sexual promiscuity and, indeed, their inability to contain their sexual urges.[76] This in turn made people pronounce themselves as judges over other people. This tendency to judge others who have already contracted HIV has not changed and things will remain that way if we continue to champion only the message of ABC at the individual level. However, this does not suggest that the ABC model is redundant. The argument here is that as far as this model focuses on an individual and ignores the African communal sexual morality, the HI virus will continue to spread. Therefore, the Seventh-day Adventist Church needs to take the above argument into consideration when dealing with the HIV and AIDS epidemic in the South African context.

Home-Based Care places pastors, trained pastoral caregivers, and volunteers in the homes of PLWHA. The introduction of Home-Based Care, which will assist the overburdened pastors and lighten their workload, requires systemic rethinking of pastoral care and social restructuring of a ministry to PLWHA from grassroots outward to the PLWHA and the larger community.

In addition to the above, the task of the Seventh-day Adventist Church in South Africa will include the starting up of communal contextual Home-Based Care programs (CHBCP) and learning[77] how to deal with stigma and discrimination, as well as how to mobilize the whole church to become a healing and caring community. This will align with its doctrine of social welfare and social health, a ministry of healing as

---

[75] Bujo (1998), 186.
[76] Ibid.
[77] "Learning" through training and teaching and the introduction of educational programs in their local churches, departments, and all Seventh-day Adventist institutions in South Africa.

elucidated by Ellen G. White,[78] a founding member of the Seventh-day Adventist Church. The Seventh-day Adventist Church holds as fundamental belief a doctrine on healthful living and lifestyle practices that reflect a theology which holds that all things must be firmly established upon the Bible. Adventists uphold a belief that a sound mind in a sound body is best able to render most effective service to God and others.[79] According to Adventist theology, care of the body—whether personally, socially, or institutionally—is fully an expression of Christian commitment. Seventh-day Adventists view the Scriptures as the major pillar of its faith that direct this doctrine of health. The Seventh-day Adventist Church has a legacy of health ministry founded upon this doctrine and shaped through the testimony of the writings of Ellen G. White known, to Seventh-day Adventists as the Spirit of Prophecy (SOP).

Seventh-day Adventists view optimal health as a God-given trust essential for day life, but also, more importantly, as essential in preparation for the second coming of Christ. The teaching of the Seventh-day Adventist Church has traditionally insisted on the integration of holistic dimensions within its congregation programs.[80] Great emphasis is placed on healthful living and lifestyle practices that avoid or abstain from all harmful foods and substances. The person who knowingly violates simple health principles, thereby bringing on illness, disease, or disability, is seen as living in violation of the laws of God.

From the early part of the 19th century, one of the pioneers of the Adventist movement, Ellen G. White, saw the need for the church to

---

[78] In brief, she was a woman of remarkable spiritual gifts who lived most of her life during the nineteenth century (1827–1915), yet through her writings she is still making a revolutionary impact on millions of people around the world. During her lifetime she wrote more than 5,000 periodical articles and forty books; but today, including compilations from her 50,000 pages of manuscripts, more than 100 titles are available in English. She is the most translated woman writer in the entire history of literature, and the most translated American author of either gender. Her writings cover a broad range of subjects, including religion, education, social relationships, evangelism, prophecy, publishing, nutrition, and management. https://1ref.us/s4 (accessed 5/6/2019).

[79] *The Seventh-day Adventist Tradition: Religious Beliefs and Healthcare Decisions*, Edited by DuBose, Edwin R; Revised by Walters, James W. Illinois (2002). https://1ref.us/s5 (accessed 5/6/2019).

[80] Okemwa (2003), 23.

embrace the holistic approach as a means of achieving its mission in the world.[81] Since then the church tradition has always looked at illness, not only as physical distress, but also as a spiritual distress, which needs to be addressed. From the Scripture point of view, the Seventh-day Adventist Church focuses on Jesus who is depicted as One who cured many diseases—helping those who were vulnerable.

Indeed, the healing of the lepers and the outcasts brought the restoration of their spiritual as well as their physical well-being, thus reinstating their human dignity and their status in the society. This shows that the Seventh-day Adventist Church in South Africa should be a place where agape love is expressed openly among its church members and PLWHA. The Seventh-day Adventist Church in South Africa finds itself in a multicultural and very diverse context. The need exists for cross-cultural healing ministries of care, and the church would do well to train its members in intercultural communication and multicultural ministries if they were to make a success of reaching the people living with HIV and AIDS through effective multi-dimensional Home-Based Care ministries. Emmanuel Lartey is of the view that the heart of the "hiddenness" of pastoral care is love.[82] Jesus, the Great Physician, ministered across class and culture in meeting the needs of the people. Therefore, as a community of faith, the Seventh-day Adventist Church should demonstrate Christ's love to all,

> "How can the Seventh-day Adventist Church engage the community of faith in pastoral care to those who are living with HIV and AIDS and how can the church initiate an effective communal contextual Home-Based Care to cater to PLWHA in poor communities?"

---

[81] Ibid.
[82] Lartey (2003), 29.

and this includes all PLWHA and all who are affected by HIV and AIDS. "We love because he first loved us" (1 John 4:19, NIV).

1.6 Reason for Choosing This Topic

My choice of this topic was partly influenced by the willingness of the Church of Sweden and the Swedish government (through the University of Stellenbosch) to finance a study of this nature. The greatest motivation for this research, however, emanates from my personal conviction that the Seventh-day Adventist Church not only has a role to play in the HIV and AIDS epidemic, but the Church also has the capacity within its structures, if effectively applied, to make remarkable contributions in responding to the AIDS crisis in South Africa. I am convinced that writing about a contextual Home-Based Care research for Seventh-day Adventists is a step forward in responding to the HIV and AIDS crisis. This written account on *HIV and AIDS as a Challenge to the Seventh-day Adventist Church in South Africa: A Reflection on Home-Based Care* could do a great deal towards facilitating a creative response in the present HIV and AIDS crisis in South Africa.

However, the implication for the Seventh-day Adventist Church in South Africa will be to do an assessment of its policy on ecclesial matters— it will be helpful to research the link between ecclesiology, the existing Seventh-day Adventist policies, if any, on HIV and AIDS, and to find a systemic, communal approach to people suffering with HIV and AIDS within poor communities.

To clarify the use of the term "ecclesiology" in this book, three dimensions are used:

1. The denominational dimension, which refers to the Seventh-day Adventist Church and its policies.
2. The Theological-Biblical dimension refers to critical discussion of text and connection to koinonia.
3. General identification of the church as the body of Christ, or the fellowship of believers.

1.7 Problem Statement

The problem statement is *"How can the Seventh-day Adventist Church engage the community of faith in pastoral care to those who are living with HIV and AIDS and how can the church initiate an effective communal contextual Home-Based Care to cater to PLWHA in poor communities?"* An investigation in answer to the problem will help us to explore how the Seventh-day Adventist Church can engage in pastoral care to the PLWHA and their families. What can help to reframe the Seventh-day Adventist Church's existing pastoral paradigms and enable them to address the challenge posed by HIV and AIDS decisively? The implication for the Seventh-day Adventist Church will be to re-visit its policy on ecclesial concerns where the spiritual and religious dimensions are examined to determine their effectiveness in caring for the sick and dying—thus the attempt to research the link between ecclesiology, the policy of the Seventh-day Adventist Church and a systemic, communal approach to people suffering with HIV and AIDS within poor communities from grassroots level, instead of the clergy only.

The core problem of this research will focus on existing policies in the Seventh-day Adventist Church. They will be critically scrutinized with the following questions in mind:

- Is the basic and fundamental ecclesiology in the Seventh-day Adventist Church with the focus on denominational and internal matters, geared and designed for a community approach with the aim to be engaged with grassroots issues pertaining to the HIV and AIDS epidemic and the needs of people in local communities to be cared for in the more intimate space of the family system and neighbourhood structures?
- What are the theological and ecclesiological implications for being the Church in poor communities with a lack of care facilities and health facilities? It is in this regard that the option of a Home-Based Care model surfaces.

- How can the Seventh-day Adventist Church restructure its current policies in order to shift the focus from a clerical model to a more community-oriented model?

With reference to the challenges of overburdened pastors, as stated earlier, with large districts and many congregations in their districts to serve and members to care for,[83] the following problems surface:

1. That pastors are carrying heavy workloads and are inundated with the varied needs of their members, including the complex and challenging needs of PLWHA both in their congregations and in the community.
2. The need now exists for pastoral leadership to share their responsibility and utilize all possible resources at their disposal to train and equip their members as caregivers and lay counsellors, etc., thus making pastoral care and counselling to PLWHA a congregational responsibility.

In the light of the above, I make the following assumptions:

- That a study of the writings and counsels of Ellen G. White on pastoral care, healthcare, and ministries to spiritually and physically sick people will be useful to prepare the lay members as volunteers in doing Home-Based Care.
- Also, a study on the important and relevant theories of Professor Daniël Louw of a pastoral hermeneutics of care and *Cura Vitae*, will prove helpful so that the Seventh-day Adventist Church in South Africa is capable of constructing a contextual Home-Based Care program that can effectively cater to the needs of the PLWHA in poor communities, and move forward from a grassroots position. Pastors, elders, and deacons, as well as caregivers in spiritual healing, will benefit greatly in receiving training in these essential tools in ministry to

---

[83] See Appendix #1: SAU Report.

PLWHA. Prof. Louw's theories provide excellent new dimensions to pastoral care and spiritual healing to the sick in our midst.

With *Cura Vitae* above is meant the following: Healing in pastoral caregiving is more extensive and comprehensive than merely an individual "soul" as in the traditional approach, namely *Cura animarum*.

With life is meant the dynamics of everyday life as determined by habitus,[84] relationships, and unpredictable happenstances. An existential approach has been developed in terms of the following six existential realities (independent from culture and geography), namely anxiety, guilt/shame, despair, helplessness/vulnerability, frustration, and anger. (See further details on *Cura Vitae* in Chapter 4.)

1.8   Basic Research Questions

1. What is the general ecclesiology of the Seventh-day Adventist Church? Is it focused more on clerical and dogmatic issues than existential life needs?
2. What kind of challenge does the HIV and AIDS epidemic put before a more operational approach/operative ecclesiology to people suffering from HIV and AIDS?
3. What is meant by a Home-Based Care model and should it be incorporated into the pastoral ministry of the Seventh-day Adventist Church?

1.9   Basic Assumptions and Presuppositions

This research is informed by the premise that the involvement and support of the Seventh-day Adventist Church in matters of HIV and AIDS is an imperative. The Seventh-day Adventist Church, therefore, is viewed as a vital organ in the community. Community health, more specifically in the context of HIV and AIDS, is an imperative to Seventh-day Adventists.

---

[84] Ingrained habits, skills, and dispositions.

Indeed, the Seventh-day Adventist Church is an integral part of the South African society, being a church equipped for more than a century now with a unique doctrine on health, Christian behavior, and conduct. In the light and revelation of health reform, the numerous departments of the worldwide Seventh-day Adventist Church, which include academic institutions, health and medical institutions, hospitals, clinics, and health centers owned and run by the church, have for decades already been instrumental in health education, disease prevention, treatment, pastoral and spiritual care, and cure. In South Africa this is no exception.

The HIV and AIDS epidemic is affecting the larger South African society especially in poor areas and churches are not spared, including the Seventh-day Adventist Church. This is because the HI virus infects and affects many of its members and many Adventists are dying of AIDS-related diseases. Therefore, the Seventh-day Adventist Church in South Africa can no longer afford to be silent and passive about the HIV and AIDS epidemic. The Seventh-day Adventist Church needs to position herself and should now empower its members in Home-Based Care projects by constructing a Home-Based Care program based on her own health message, their doctrine on social health wellness, and their teachings on medical missionaries as taught by Ellen G. White. However, her pastoral approach will not be contextual unless an intercultural model is taken into consideration.[85] The Seventh-day Adventist Church now needs to structure Home-Based Care projects where "care is given in the home of the person living with HIV and AIDS, ... supported by a trained community caregiver, ... and where the team of caregivers consists of all the

> *"The Seventh-day Adventist Church is an integral part of the South African society, being a church equipped for more than a century now with a unique doctrine on health, Christian behavior, and conduct."*

---

[85] Lartey (1997), 30.

people involved in care and support, and may include a medical practitioner or professional nurse, or trained counsellor, a pastor or spiritual counsellor and volunteers" that will ensure that the poor PLWHA will experience the benefits and blessings of healing and care in their communities where they live.[86]

1.10 Objectives of This Research

1. The core objective of this research is to formulate a contextual Home-Based Care program within the Seventh-day Adventist Church in South Africa. The statistics discussed earlier revealed that the majority of PLWHA live among the poor in the country. The Seventh-day Adventist Church is to explore providing a structure or program, the resources and framework, that will enable the family of PLWHA to look after their own sick members. Therefore, the focus will also be on de-stigmatization, support of families of PLWHA, educating the community about prevention of HIV transmission, and to bring the presence of God into the homes of PLWHA in poor communities through compassionate Home-Based Care programs. In this way poor communities and families of PLWHA will be empowered to cope effectively with the physical, psychological, and spiritual needs of PLWHA.
2. Secondly, the aim is to show how the core concepts of health and a ministry of healing can be used by the Seventh-day Adventist Church to mobilize their local resources needed for socio-economic empowerment of the PLWHA and their families. This is useful when constructing a communal, contextual Home-Based Care Program (HBCP) modelled on principles of health and well-being. The understanding of the interplay between poverty and the HIV and AIDS epidemic, which is a reality in Africa, is crucial. The Seventh-day Adventist Church needs to put structures and programs in place to care for the PLWHA in the communities where they live.

---

[86] Van Dyk (2008), 332.

3. Thirdly, the aim is to show how the Seventh-day Adventist Church can interculturate her pastoral strategies so as to respond effectively to the challenge posed by the HIV and AIDS epidemic. Prior to a unified church in 2005 in South Africa, the different races had separate conferences that operated independently caring for their members. Now that the church has been merged into one conference since 2005, the need for training in intercultural competencies in ministry and pastoral care are vital so that pastors and caregivers can effectively cater and care for all race groups among their memberships.
4. Finally, the aim is to demonstrate how the Seventh-day Adventist Church can mobilize her members in effective ministries to PLWHA by becoming volunteers in the contextual Home-Based Care program. Every believer a volunteer means that every church member is a volunteer in caring for PLWHA and their families. This means that the church needs to train them adequately for the challenges posed by the HIV and AIDS epidemic. It is interesting to examine the interplay between Seventh-day Adventist spirituality and African spirituality, and how both of these can help us understand health and healing in the context of the HIV and AIDS epidemic, thus engaging the church more actively and in successful ministries to PLWHA. This will therefore involve an intercultural model.[87]

1.11 Theoretical Framework

This research is based on a theoretical framework founded on pastoral hermeneutics as demonstrated by Prof. Daniël Louw in his book, *A Pastoral Hermeneutics of Care and Encounter: A Theological Design for a Basic Theory, Anthropology, Method and Therapy*. This hermeneutics of pastoral theology is focused on textual and contextual metaphors, symbols, language, and narratives that provide healing, change, transformation, care, service, and help. It fosters the rediscovering of our human identity

---

[87] Lartey (1997), 30.

before God, while simultaneously articulating the re-discovering of the "you" in the "me," and through an empathic pastoral endeavor putting oneself in the place of another person. In a ministry to PLWHA one should try to put oneself in someone else's shoes. This pastoral venture deems the promissory character of the biblical texts as essential, because a daily encounter with biblical texts, especially as vehicles of address from God, are able to transform our human quest for meaning in accordance with the creativity of divine promise.[88] Not only am I a former student of Prof. Daniël Louw, but have applied his theories in clinical and practical work done in hospices and centers that cater to PLWHA, where I have seen how his theological design will definitely enhance an understanding of how the Seventh-day Adventist Church should embrace an intercultural model and hence formulate a contextual Home-Based Care program modelled for the South African context. The dynamics of pastoral hermeneutics bring the presence of God the Great Healer to where PLWHA find themselves and provide pastors with excellent tools in care and encounter with God.

1.12   Methodology

The methodology of this research study is non-empirical.

1. It is a literature research and critical analysis of existing documents of the Seventh-day Adventist Church. The research work required consultation of written sources on the denominational history of the Seventh-day Adventist Church in South Africa, its education, and advocacies on health. It will be a critical assessment of data. I have consulted books, journals, articles, and other relevant documents related to the research topic. It is therefore also a qualitative research: making an assessment of the current documents in the Seventh-day Adventist Church on health care and health issues related to the

---

[88] Louw (2005), 107.

research topic of HIV and AIDS intervention in South Africa in order to meet the objectives of this research.
2. It is a hermeneutical approach, thus the attempt to scrutinize existing texts and documents of the Seventh-day Adventist Church, with the following question in mind: How should they be linked to the context of people suffering from HIV and AIDS, and what is the potential impact their implementation could have in this crisis?
3. Furthermore, it is a logical reasoning and reflection:
   a) Theological reflection
   b) Religious reflection
   c) Ecclesiological reflection
4. It is also a participatory observation: My personal experience in the fields of theology, education, and HIV and AIDS intervention, as well as personal involvement at J.L. Zwane and Ihkwezi Clinic, played a vital role in the writing of this research. Furthermore, I am a person of Seventh-day Adventist persuasion and one who knows the history of the Seventh-day Adventist Church in South Africa. Throughout the book hermeneutical tools will be used to interpret various phenomena or contexts.

1.13 Scope and Limitations

This research is limited to the Seventh-day Adventist Church in South Africa with the focus on Home-Based Care to PLWHA.

1.14 Structure and Outline

This book is divided into four chapters:

i) In **Chapter One** the general background and overview of the important aspects of this research are presented. The aims and research question are presented. The HIV and AIDS scenario in the South African context is explored, as well as the challenge facing the

Seventh-day Adventist Church in South Africa. In addition, the basic assumptions, research presuppositions, methodology, and objectives are also highlighted.

ii) **Chapter Two** will serve as an introduction to the Seventh-day Adventist Church in South Africa and its administrative structure. The current policies of the Seventh-day Adventist Church on HIV and AIDS will be discussed, and health and healing within SDA spirituality will be explored. Here the focus will also be on the notion of important pillars of the Seventh-day Adventist faith that can enhance a ministry to PLWHA, with the Scriptures as the most important pillar to Seventh-day Adventists, the role and function of Seventh-day Adventist departments and institutions, and the challenge that the church faces in the South African context.

iii) In **Chapter Three** the HIV and AIDS epidemic as a challenge to existing ecclesiologies: towards an eclectic contextual Home-Based Care in the Seventh-day Adventist Church, will be a general investigation on how the HIV and AIDS epidemic challenges traditional understanding of the Christian church as an institution. Study is given to the hierarchical and clerical models with the emphasis on the role of official clergy.

iv) In **Chapter Four** there will be an attempt to formulate a theory for pastoral care and counselling to PLWHA and their families within the Seventh-day Adventist Church context. The SDA model of contextual Home-Based Care programs to PLWHA will be discussed. The chapter deals with how the Seventh-day Adventist Church can model its Home-Based Care programs in the South African context and how it can mobilize its members to support the HBC projects. A pastoral strategy will be provided and the potential of the pillars of Adventist faith in healing the PLWHA and their families will be examined. Finally, recommendations and/or suggestions of a way forward for Seventh-day Adventists in South Africa will be discussed.

1.15 Conclusion

The research background, statement of the problem, the basic assumptions and presuppositions, scope, and the limitations of the research, as well as research objectives, theoretical framework, research methodology, and the chapter outline is presented in this chapter.

The background for exploring how the Seventh-day Adventist Church in South Africa can construct a contextual Home-Based Care program is also given. Before we come to that it is crucial to introduce the reader to the Seventh-day Adventist Church in South Africa and to examine health and healing within the context of Seventh-day Adventist spirituality.

CHAPTER TWO

Introduction to the Seventh-day Adventist Church: Structure and Current Policies of the Church on HIV and AIDS

2.1 History of the Seventh-day Adventist Church in South Africa

This chapter serves as an introduction to the background and development of the Seventh-day Adventist Church in South Africa and its administrative structure. It will also focus on the notion of important pillars within the doctrines of the Seventh-day Adventist faith that would be helpful in the formation of a contextual Home-Based Care program and the challenge that the church faces in the South African context. Furthermore, it will be a critical analysis of the policies of the Seventh-day Adventist Church on HIV and AIDS, its impact on current ecclesial structures, and to investigate ways in which the Seventh-day Adventist Church structures their ministry to PLWHA based on their doctrine of healthcare and well-being, which is imperative to a Home-Based Care ministry.

2.2 Background

This introduction to the history and background of the Seventh-day Adventist Church in South Africa does not intend to convey any tone of finality. This chapter will mainly be descriptive to provide the reader with insights into the structure and development of the church organization and the rapid advancement of the work in the country. It has been quite challenging to find or access completed works on the comprehensive history of the Seventh-day Adventist Church in South Africa, for this paper revealed the need for a more accurate and comprehensive[89] history than is currently available. There is a need for the history of the Seventh-day Adventist Church in South Africa to be documented from the time of its inception, to preserve its heritage in written form,[90] and to make it available for tertiary use[91] as well. This research therefore mainly relied on archival materials accessed at the Ellen G. White Research Institute located at Helderberg College, Somerset West, South Africa, where the main documents on the early history are held.

The worldwide Seventh-day Adventist Church has its roots in the Great Awakening, which took place mainly in the United States of America in the 1840s. The name of the church organization, "*Seventh-day*

---

[89] Given the political history in South Africa, where apartheid formed a significant part of its history, the Seventh-day Adventist Church in South Africa, until recently, also practiced separatism, that is, separate administrative conferences for Blacks, Whites, Indians, and Coloureds (du Preez, 2010, 316), and therefore they each have their own historic backgrounds (story) and developments. The author had difficulty in obtaining a reliable comprehensive written history.

[90] "The most natural divisions of time for the historical background and development of the SDA Church in Southern Africa fall into three periods:

1920–1931: 1920 when the African Division of Seventh-day Adventists was organized, to 1931, when it was reorganized under the name Southern Africa Division;

1931–1945: Covering the years of the Great Depression and World War II;

1946–1960: The Post-war period" (Thompson, 1977). RCL, PHD dissertation Introduction.

[91] Dr Gerald du Preez in his last three of six recommendations of his Doctor of Philosophy dissertation:

#Recommendation 4: That further research is undertaken in order to provide a comprehensive general history of the SDA Church in South Africa and that this be published for use in the tertiary and general reading arena;

#Recommendation 5: That research into the Black Church in South Africa be engaged in to ensure that that segment of history is not lost to posterity;

#Recommendation 6: That students, amateur historians, church members, and church leaders give serious attention and study to recording and preserving the history of individual pioneers, congregations, and institutions—the culture of history needs to be cultivated and nurtured to ensure that future generations will have landmarks and monuments that can testify to God's leading in His Church (du Preez, 2010).

Adventist Church,"⁹² was adopted in 1860. Then only later the Seventh-day Adventist Church was officially organized and registered in 1863.⁹³ At the time of formal registration the total membership of the Seventh-day Adventist church was 3,500, all of which lived in North America, with 125 churches and five conferences. The ministers numbered twenty-two ordained and eight licensed.⁹⁴ The work of the Church was mainly confined to the United States of America but there was some interest in various parts of the world. We find that an interesting combination of events brought its missionaries eventually to South Africa in the last quarter of the century. In 1874 the first foreign missionary to be sent out by the Church was a man by the name of J. N. Andrews, to Europe. In the same year the Seventh-day Adventist Church also established their first institution of higher education, a college, in Battle Creek, Michigan, USA. And by 1901 the Church had already laid the foundation for its rapid expansion in the 20th century. At the time the Seventh-day Adventist Church already had a very strong education system in place. Sanitariums, hospitals, and clinics in many parts of the world marked its well-established medical missionary work. The Church also established several publishing houses in many different parts of the world. By that time Seventh-day Adventists had developed an organizational system that still serves the Church today, and had a strong mission program in many parts of the world.⁹⁵

---

⁹² The name Seventh-day Adventist carries the true features of our faith in front and will convict the inquiring mind. Like an arrow from the Lord's quiver, it will wound the transgressor of God's Law, and will lead to repentance toward God and faith in our Lord Jesus Christ (White, *Testimonies for the Church, Vol. 1*, 224).

⁹³ The first general official gathering of Seventh-day Adventists was held at Battle Creek, Michigan, in 1863. A constitution of nine articles was adopted. These articles have been added to at subsequent sessions (*Church Heritage*: 30).

⁹⁴ *Church Heritage*, 30.

⁹⁵ Birkenstock (2004).

2.3 Origin of the Seventh-day Adventists in South Africa

2.3.1 Men and Movements in the 1800s

According to Birkenstock, "In many parts of the world, men and movements arose during the 19th century that focused on the fulfilment of prophecy that related to the Second Advent of Christ by 1844." This was not the case in South Africa. Whereas many mission stations were started during the 1800s in South Africa by many different mission societies, there were no major movements that took place. In South Africa the origins of the Seventh-day Adventist Church were due to spontaneous understandings of the Bible by certain Dutch people living in the Free State and Cape provinces, and later, by English farmers in the Eastern Cape.

2.3.2 Pieter Johannes Daniel Wessels

Apparently, a man by the name of Pieter Wessels played a very significant part in the early stages of Adventists in South Africa. He was born in February 1856, one of fifteen children from two marriages. He was a serious young boy who was confused about why there were so many different churches and by the age of fourteen he asked his mother which was the right church. She told him to believe the Bible. So, at the age of twenty-one years of age, he concluded his own theory: "Either the Bible is right and all the Churches wrong, because of the so many churches, or the Churches are right and the Bible is wrong." Wessels lived on his farm Osfontein near Kimberley, where he provided milk and vegetables to the mine diggers at the diamond fields. In the early 1880s an American faith healer visited the Free State and preached in

> *"Either the Bible is right and all the Churches wrong, because of the so many churches, or the Churches are right and the Bible is wrong."*

Andrew Murray's church. Philip Wessels, the brother of Pieter Wessels, after attending and listening, became convinced of "Prayer Healing" and shared his convictions with his brother, Pieter. Soon after this, Pieter contracted pneumonia and when his wife and his mother wanted to call in a doctor, Pieter refused. He said that God could heal him in answer to prayer—he prayed and the next day he was healed. He promised God that if He healed him, he would follow all that the Bible teaches.

2.3.3   Pieter Wessels Decided to Keep the Seventh-day Sabbath

As a next step after this change, Pieter wanted to convince his brother Johannes about faith healing. So in response to this his brother Johannes told him that if he really wanted to be religious, why does he not keep the Sabbath of the Bible, which is Saturday, the seventh day of the week? Johannes showed him that the Sabbath has been changed to the first day of the week. Upon Pieter's study about this change, he became convinced that Saturday is the seventh day and that he needed to keep the seventh-day Sabbath. So, on Saturday 26th November 1885, he kept the Sabbath and believed that he was the only person in the whole world keeping the Sabbath.

2.3.4   George Van Druten Accepts the Seventh-day Sabbath

Apparently, around the same time, another farmer living in the Boshoff by the name of George Van Druten came to the same conclusion about the Sabbath. When one of his children became seriously ill, he prayed for guidance about where to go for medical help—whether to go to Kimberley or Bloemfontein. After loading his family into the buggy, they headed for the main road, which was where they would need to decide which way to turn. Apparently this was where he became aware of a horseman just ahead and felt impressed to follow—the horseman took the road that lead to Bloemfontein, and then strangely disappeared. This was totally flat countryside, and yet the horseman simply disappeared. Before midnight he outspanned as he refused to travel on the Sabbath, Sunday, and planned to continue the journey the following night after the Sabbath. Despite his wife's pleadings, Van Druten would not budge. During the night he had a dream about a man who asked him why he was so troubled. In response to this he replied that his child was ill and that he was not willing to travel on the Sabbath. The man in the dream asked which day was the Sabbath. He said that that the fourth commandment said the seventh day. The "Man" then said that Sunday was not the seventh day. To Van Druten's shock and horror he discovered that Sunday was the first day. So on Sunday Van Druten continued his journey and the first thing he did was to pay a visit to his minister, Andrew Murray, residing in Bloemfontein. When Andrew Murray had difficulty in explaining who changed the days, George Van Druten approached a Jewish Rabbi who said that the Law was immutable and confirmed that Saturday, the seventh day, was the Sabbath. Van Druten then spoke to Pieter Wessels. They thought that they were the only two people with convictions about Saturday, as the seventh-day Sabbath.

2.3.5 George Van Druten and William Hunt

Shortly after this Van Druten moved to a farm near Kimberley called Alexandersfontein. One Saturday afternoon he was walking past the huts of the diggers. He noticed a man dressed in his Sunday best sitting in front of his hut and not working but reading his Bible instead. Upon their meeting, George Van Druten discovered that William Hunt was a Seventh-day Adventist. Hunt was a fortune seeker from California who came to the diamond fields. About one month after Van Druten discovered the true Bible Sabbath from Bible study, he visited Pieter Wessels. He told Wessels that a miner from Nevada (USA) named William Hunt was also keeping the Seventh-day Sabbath. Wessels wrote November 17, 1924, "Brother Van Druten handed me a copy of the *Review and Herald* which he had received from Brother Hunt. Brother Van Druten reported that William Hunt said there were 30,000 Sabbath keepers in America." Pieter Wessels then also was introduced to William Hunt who in turn put them in touch with the Seventh-day Adventist Church in the United States of America. Eager to know more Bible truth, together Wessels and Van Druten then wrote to the headquarters in America and appealed to the General Conference for a Dutch minister to come teach them more fully and to baptize them. They sent along fifty pounds, which was the equivalent of two hundred and fifty dollars, to defray expenses. "This was the 1886 *'Macedonian Call'* from South Africa. When this letter was read at the 1886 General Conference Session in the Battle Creek Tabernacle, its message electrified the assembled delegates who rose and sang the doxology."[96] The story of these two men spread rapidly among the locals and soon a number of families joined them in keeping Saturday, the seventh-day Sabbath.

2.3.6 The First Missionaries Arrive in South Africa in July 1887

In July 1887, the first five missionaries arrived in the Cape from America to organize the Church in South Africa. These were the two ministers, D. A. Robinson and C. L. Boyd with their wives; and two colporteurs, George Burleigh and R. S. Antony; and Miss Carrie Mace, a Bible Instructor. At that time Pastor Robinson remained in the Cape, while Pastor Boyd proceeded to the diamond fields, where he found about forty adults, including a number of children, keeping the seventh-day Sabbath.

2.3.7 Organization of the Seventh-day Adventist Church in South Africa

According to Birkenstock, Boyd travelled to Beaconsfield in Kimberley to organize the first Seventh-day Adventist congregation there and by 14 May 1890 they had their first church building. The first Seventh-day Adventist church building in South Africa, made of wood and iron, was erected in Beaconsfield, a suburb of Kimberley. Today this church building stands as a national monument as the first Seventh-day Adventist

---

[96] *Church Heritage*, 36, 37.

church in South Africa. The second church building, which was the first Seventh-day Adventist church in the Cape Peninsula, was erected in Roeland Street, Cape Town.

In Cape Town, D. A. Robinson began his ministry by giving lectures on non-doctrinal subjects in various churches. Colporteurs sold copies of studies of *Daniel and Revelation* by Uriah Smith. In January 1888, a tent, sent from America, was pitched in a sheltered spot in Claremont, a suburb of Cape Town, for evangelistic meetings. The preacher was Ira I. Hankins. As a result of evangelistic outreach in this tent, the second congregation in South Africa was organized (established) in Claremont, Cape Town. The third congregation to be organized was the Rokeby Park Church in the Eastern Cape. Then contacts were made with Wessels at Kimberley by transport wagons from the Eastern Cape by men called Pastors Tarr and Davies. When they returned to Bathurst others also joined the church—Hankins, Staples, Willmores, and Sparrows—these all played an important role in the expansion of the Church in South Africa.

2.3.8 The Cape became the Headquarters of the SDA Church in South Africa

The Cape became the headquarters of the Seventh-day Adventist Church for its activities in South Africa. The Wessels family were a very wealthy family. They sold their farm in Kimberley, with its diamonds on it, to the De Beers Company and with those proceeds they assisted the Church in establishing various enterprises and to acquire a number of buildings.

2.4 Important Pillars in the Seventh-day Adventist Faith

2.4.1 Education and Institutions of Learning

Education is one of the significant hallmarks of Seventh-day Adventists, and also of significant importance to the subject of this book. The Seventh-day Adventist Church has a unique philosophy of education and therefore they place an enormous emphasis on a sound education program that is based on the principles of their Adventist philosophy of education. Wherever there is an Adventist presence, it is encouraged that Adventist schools and institutions of higher education are established to provide its members, their families, and the community with a solid Christian education. Seventh-day Adventists believe that to educate is to redeem. The main goal of Adventist education, therefore, is to restore the image of God in all students, a redemptive purpose that encompasses Seventh-day Adventist and non-Seventh-day Adventist students alike.

Claremont Union College, the first Seventh-day Adventist College outside of the United States of America, was founded in Claremont, near Kenilworth, Cape Town, South Africa, in 1892 and became officially operational in 1893. Today the building is a national monument which forms part of a shopping mall on Rosmead Avenue, Claremont. The college was in operation from 1893–1917. Later, Spioenkop College (1919–1927) was built near Ladysmith, Natal.[97] Then in 1928 the Helderberg College in Somerset West was established and is still fully functioning today.[98] The library on the Helderberg College campus, the Pieter Wessels Library, was named after the Wessels family who had invested extensively in the funding and establishment of the university and campus facilities.

2.4.2 Printing and Publishing

Similarly, since the early inception of the Church in South Africa, Seventh-day Adventists invested largely in printing and publishing establishments. On 14 February 1916, the Sentinel Publishing Company was established also on Rosmead Avenue, Kenilworth, Cape Town. The publishing company was moved to Bloemfontein in 2000 and was fully operational in

---

[97] *Church Heritage*, 40.
[98] Helderberg College, a SAQA (South African Qualifications Authority) accredited university which is located in Helderberg, Somerest West, Cape Town, is also the Alma Mater of the author, where she completed a bachelor's degree in theology (1998–2001) in preparation for pastoral ministry.

2001 at the premises of the Southern African Union, headquarters of the Seventh-day Adventist Church in South Africa.

2.4.3 Sanitariums and Medical Facilities

Of primary importance to this subject and significant to education in an HIV and AIDS ministry, is the early establishment of medical facilities owned and run by Seventh-day Adventists since the late 1800s. The most ambitious project of all that the Church established was the well-functioning Claremont sanitarium[99] modelled after the Battle Creek sanitarium[100] in the United States of America. The sanitarium was very popular and well supported, and according to Birkenstock, even Louis Botha[101] went there for treatment. Soon after the Anglo Boer war the sanitarium was burnt to the ground. A second one was built, but in 1920 it ceased in its operations.[102] The medical missionary work, health centers, and the establishment of facilities of care play an important role in a ministry and service to PLWHA.

2.4.4 The Seventh-day Adventist Church and Mission Endeavors

Outreach endeavors were made to Rhodesia[103] upon which the Solusi Mission station became the first of its kind. Cecil John Rhodes gifted the

---

[99] CLAREMONT SANITARIUM (CLAREMONT/CAPETOWN, ZA). A fifty-one-room medical institution operated from 1897 to 1905 near Claremont, a suburb of Cape Town, South Africa, under the direction of the International Medical Missionary and Benevolent Association of Battle Creek Michigan (the organization headed by J. H. Kellogg). No expense was spared to make it the best-equipped medical institution south of the equator, the total cost amounting to £50,000, of which the Wessels family contributed £30,000. The first medical director was R. S. Anthony, M.D. (a former pioneer colporteur), who was later assisted by Kate Lindsay, M.D., who came from Battle Creek Sanitarium. Within a week of opening, every bed was filled and it became necessary to rent adjacent buildings. However, early in 1920, the sanitarium ceased in its operations. From the *Seventh-day Adventist Encyclopedia*. Published with permission from the Review and Herald Publishing Association.

[100] Dr J. H. Kellogg, founder of the Kellogg Foundation, was the first Medical Superintendent of the Battle Creek Sanitarium.

[101] First Prime Minister of the Union of South Africa.

[102] Birkenstock, E. G. White Estate.

[103] Currently known as Zimbabwe.

Seventh-day Adventist Church with 1,200 acres of land via Dr. Jameson. Today, the Solusi University in Zimbabwe, then known as Rhodesia, is still fully in operation. It was the work of pioneer W. A. Anderson who established mission stations, mission schools, and colleges in Angola, Congo, Rwanda, Burundi, Zimbabwe, Malawi, East Africa, and all parts of Africa. Many graduates from Helderberg College were sent out as missionaries to different countries in Africa, until South Africa became isolated from Africa and the rest of the world in 1960 and onwards.

2.5 The Seventh-day Adventist Church Organization

2.5.1 The Hierarchical Structure of the Seventh-day Adventist Church Organization

Generally, the Seventh-day Adventist Church operates on a hierarchical structure. The chart of the organizational structure of the Seventh-day Adventist Church presented here in Figure 1 gives a brief overview of the hierarchical structure of the church government. This helps provide background to understand the roles of the General Conference and the Southern Africa Union as they seek to address the HIV and AIDS epidemic.

2.5.2 The Seventh-day Adventist Church Organization as at 2004

By 2004 the General Conference, world headquarters of the Seventh-day Adventist Church, was located in Silver Spring, Maryland, USA, in the Washington D.C. district. At the time the Seventh-day Adventist Church had members living in 203 of the 228 countries recognized by the United Nations Organization, with a world Church membership exceeding 14,000,000 members. The world Church was divided into thirteen divisions. Divisions were divided into unions and by 2004 there were a total of ninety-four unions. Unions are divided into conferences, missions, and fields. Pastors are appointed to districts made up of local congregations. Districts in turn form part of regions that fall under the conference.[104]

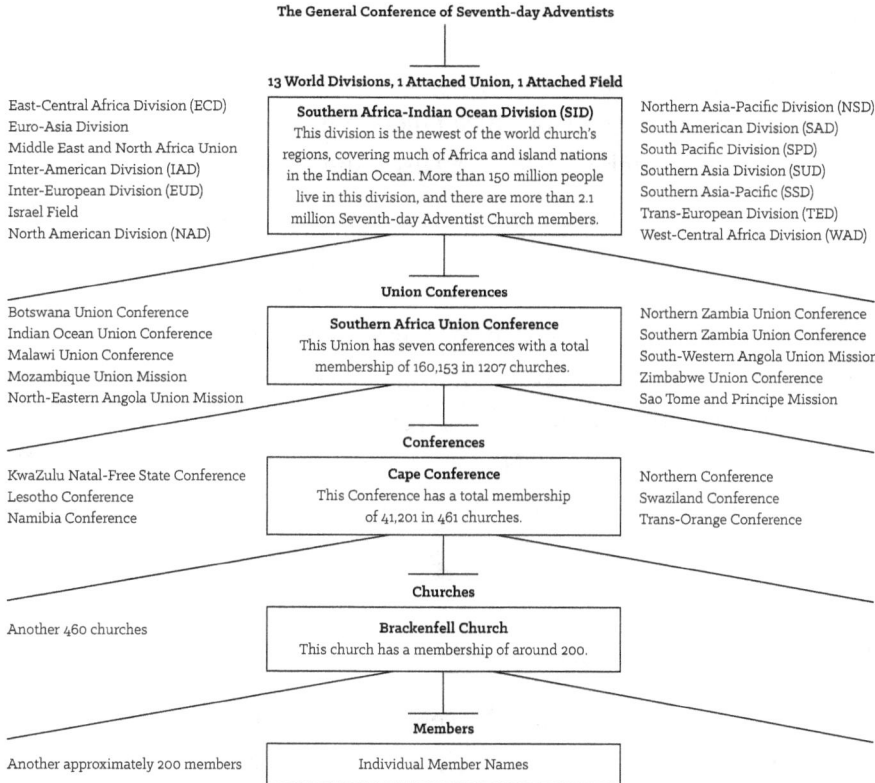

Figure 1: Organizational Structure of the Seventh-day Adventist Church

---

[104] Currently the global membership of the SDA Church exceeds 18,000,000 (eighteen million). The Seventh-day Adventist Church, one of the fastest-growing Christian movements in the world, has recorded over eighteen million baptized members. As of September 30, 2013, according to the Church's Archives, Statistics, and Research Department, there were 18,028,796 Seventh-day Adventists worldwide. December 17, 2013: According to G. T. Du Preez, Ministerial Director of the SAU, the current membership in the Southern Africa Union is 156,269.

Adventist Review Online: https://1ref.us/s6 (accessed 5/6/2019).

2.6 Main Areas of Work of the Worldwide SDA Church and Institutions by 2004

2.6.1 Education

By 2002 the worldwide Seventh-day Adventist Church had 6,355 schools and institutions of learning of which ninety-nine were colleges and universities with a total number of students exceeding 1,200,000.

2.6.2 Health

Health and healthcare facilities owned and run by the Seventh-day Adventist Church: 169 sanitariums and hospitals; 393 clinics and dispensaries; 128 nursing homes and retirement centers; thirty-three orphanages—these all with more than 10,000,000 outpatient visits in the year 2002. By 2002 the Seventh-day Adventist Church also operated twenty-seven health food industries.

2.6.3 Humanitarian Work

By 2002 ADRA, the Adventist Development and Relief Agency, operational in disaster-stricken areas worldwide, had extended its humanitarian work to 125 countries around the world. In that year alone its disaster relief and development projects directly benefited over 16,000,000 people at a cost of over $18,000,000.[105]

2.6.4 Publishing Work

By 2002 the Seventh-day Adventist Church was already operating fifty-seven publishing houses around the world, printing in 338 different languages, and running programs around the world using 834 languages and dialects.

---

[105] https://1ref.us/s7 (accessed 35/6/2019).

2.6.5 Missionary Work

Although most of the work of the Seventh-day Adventist Church is done by the leaders in their local churches, by 2002 it had more than 500 missionaries used for their specialist services in particular areas of the world, for example, health, education, development, etc.

2.7 Other Services of the Seventh-day Adventist Church

- Adventist Television Network—The Hope TV channel is the official TV network for the denomination running religious and health programs.[106]
- AWR: Adventist World Radio serving various parts of the world via short wave radio for spreading the gospel.[107]
- Christian Record Services for the Blind.[108]
- Geoscience Research Institute.[109]
- Institute of World Mission.[110]
- Ellen G. White Research Centers.[111]
- Biblical Research Institute.[112]
- Global Mission Centers—Buddhist/Hindu/Islamic/Jewish/Urban secular study centers.[113]

---

[106] https://1ref.us/s8 (accessed 5/6/2019).
[107] https://1ref.us/s9 (accessed 5/6/2019).
[108] https://1ref.us/sa (accessed 5/6/2019).
[109] https://1ref.us/sb (accessed 5/6/2019).
[110] https://1ref.us/sc (accessed 5/6/2019).
[111] https://1ref.us/sd (accessed 5/6/2019); https://1ref.us/sf (accessed 5/6/2019). There are also others around the world. These are two examples.
[112] https://1ref.us/sg (accessed 5/6/2019).
[113] https://1ref.us/sh (accessed 5/6/2019).

2.8 The Seventh-day Adventist Church in South Africa as at 2004

The headquarters of the Southern African Union is located in Bloemfontein. At 2004 the Seventh-day Adventist Church in the Southern African Union had a membership reaching over the 90,000 mark in 733 churches throughout South Africa. There are eight conferences and fields throughout the country, each with its own headquarters. According to Pastor Gerald du Preez, Ministerial Director of the SAU, the current church membership in the Southern Africa Union is at 156,269 in 2015.

2.8.1 Education

> "Education is regarded as a pillar in the Seventh-day Adventist faith."

Education is regarded as a pillar in the Seventh-day Adventist faith. The Church in South Africa has eleven schools, including two universities: Helderberg College in Somerset West and Bethel College in Butterworth.

2.8.2 Hospitals and Healthcare Facilities

Seventh-day Adventists own and run one hospital, five clinics and dispensaries, and eighteen nursing homes and retirement centers.

2.8.3 Humanitarian Works

ADRA, Adventist Disaster and Relief Agency, centers are in operation in various parts of the country.

2.8.4 Printing and Publishing

The Southern Publishing Association, previously called The Sentinel Publishing Company, which is now situated in Bloemfontein at the

Headquarters, takes care of all the official printing of religious materials, books, Bible study guides, and evangelistic materials of the Seventh-day Adventist Church in South Africa.

2.8.5 Voice of Prophecy Bible Correspondence School

The Seventh-day Adventist Church in South Africa operates a Bible Correspondence School located in Claremont, Cape Town, which offers free correspondence Bible study courses to the broader community. It had more than 20,000 students throughout South Africa and beyond by 2004.

2.9 The Seventh-day Adventist Doctrine on Health

> It also means that because our bodies are the temples of the Holy Spirit, we are to care for them intelligently. Along with adequate exercise and rest, we are to adopt the most healthful diet possible and abstain from the unclean foods identified in the Scriptures. Since alcoholic beverages, tobacco, and the irresponsible use of drugs and narcotics are harmful to our bodies, we are to abstain from them as well.[114]

One of the strongest pillars in Adventism is their message and emphasis on the doctrine of holistic health and healing, and healthful living as a lifestyle to maintain alongside spirituality. This doctrine of health is of utmost importance to me because of my personal beliefs on healthful living. I have gained significant insights on health and healthcare methods for the sick over years of study. This doctrine of health is also significantly important in nature as a great contribution to this research and the study on Home-Based Care to PLWHA for the following reasons: I am trained

---

[114] Vow No. 10, Fundamental Belief No. 22: Christian Behavior, https://1ref.us/tc (accessed 5/6/2019).

and have gained skill in Home-Based Care and counselling of PLWHA. I am also a member of the Seventh-day Adventist Church who is qualified in the field of theology and am a pastor who has years of experience in pastoral care and counselling, and working with terminally ill members in the community, including PLWHA and their families. Because of first-hand experience and success stories in pastoral care as healthcare ministry, I am of the opinion that the century-old proven benefits and advantages of the principles of health as taught by the Seventh-day Adventist Church, as well as their healthcare methods and advocacies on medical missionary work, are the answer to the HIV and AIDS epidemic and therefore a worthwhile contribution for treatment and care of PLWHA in South Africa.

As pointed out earlier, the Seventh-day Adventist Church holds as a pillar of their faith the doctrine on health based on the teachings of Ellen G. White that,

> Christ gave a perfect representation of true godliness by combining the work of a physician and a minister, ministering to the needs of both body and soul, healing physical disease, and then speaking words that brought peace to the troubled heart. Christ has empowered his church to do the same work that he did during his ministry.[115]

The genius of the Seventh-day Adventist health message is in the combining of both gospel and medical ministry together. It treats the patient as a whole person who needs healing of body, mind, and soul. There is a close relationship between body and mind. In order to promote the clarity of mind necessary for the comprehension of spiritual things, the laws of health must be heeded. Yet, there is great healing power in the peace that attends those who entrust themselves to the care of the Great Physician.[116]

---

[115] White, *Review and Herald*, June 9, 1904.

[116] "We should ever remember that the efficiency of the medical missionary work is in pointing sin-sick men and women to the Man of Calvary, who taketh away the sin of the world. By beholding

To meet people at the point where they know they have a need opens them up to the other aspects of well-being and health that bring a full, well-rounded life within reach. In most cases Seventh-day Adventist pastors are trained in basic health care and ministry to those who are sick and the suffering.

> The Lord ... did not wish the medical missionary work to be separated from the gospel work, or the gospel work separated from the medical missionary work. These are to blend. The medical missionary work is to be regarded as the pioneer work. It is to be the means of breaking down prejudice. As the right arm, it is to open doors for the gospel message.[117]
>
> ...Christ's ministers must stand in an altogether different position. They must be evangelists; they [also] must be medical missionaries. They must take hold of the work intelligently. But it is of no use for them to think that they can do this while they drop the work which God has said should be connected with the gospel. If they drop out the medical missionary work, they need not think that they can carry forward their work successfully, for they have only half the necessary facilities.[118]

---

him they will be changed into his likeness. Our object in establishing sanitariums is to encourage the sick and suffering to look to Jesus and live. Let the workers in our medical institutions keep Christ, the Great Physician, constantly before those to whom disease of body and soul has brought discouragement. Point them to the One who can heal both physical and spiritual diseases. Tell them of the One who is touched with the feeling of their infirmities. Encourage them to place themselves in the care of him who gave his life to make it possible for them to have life eternal. Keep their minds fixed upon the One altogether lovely, the Chiefest among ten thousand. Talk of his love; tell of his power to save" (White, *Counsels on Health*, 528.2).

[117] White, *Manuscript Releases, Vol. 13*, 203.4.
[118] White, *Manuscript Releases, Vol. 13*, 206.

Sound counsel is given to the Seventh-day Adventist Church that "The ministry and the medical missionary work must be combined. Never lose sight of this."[119]

As the medical missionary work and gospel ministry are united, they keep each other in balance. The resources available for the work can be used to establish a well-rounded ministry to minister to the whole person. On the one hand, the danger in separating them from each other includes competition for resources rather than a balanced, harmonious work. On the other hand, the beneficiaries of these ministries are desperately in need of a holistic approach, whether they realize it or not. Their sense of need creates an opportunity to lead them to the feet of the Great Physician who not only makes effective the healing remedies He has created and specified, but who will also heal them from the disease of soul that all too often underlies their illness. A medical work without gospel ministry relieves the sufferer's sense of need without leading them to the necessary and fuller healing of soul as well as body. All too often they then turn away from the fountain of life.[120]

However, given the South African context with the country being the world capital in HIV infections, the need for pastoral care is far greater than the local district pastors can cope with.

2.10 Adventist Healthcare Ministries and Home-Based Care—"Mi-Yittan!"

Having stated the counsel of Ellen G. White above, that in instances where the ministers fail to care for the sick, the work of gospel ministry cannot

---

[119] White, Letter 40 (1899), Feb. 23, para. 37.

[120] "The medical missionary work should be a part of the work of every church in our land. Disconnected from the church, it would soon become a strange medley of disorganized atoms. It would consume, but not produce. Instead of acting as God's helping hand to forward His truth, it would sap the life and force from the church and weaken the message. Conducted independently, it would not only consume talent and means needed in other lines, but in the very work of helping the helpless apart from the ministry of the word, it would place men where they would scoff at Bible truth" (White, *Counsels on Health*, 514.1).

move forward. In instances where a spirit of apathy and attitudes of indifference prevail among the Seventh-day Adventist ministers when it comes to a ministry to PLWHA, the cry of *"Mi-Yittan"* must go out. While many pastors in South Africa complain about the scores of funerals they conduct and the sick among their members, it appears as though their interests lean more strongly towards jostling for position and ambition to save the church as an organization—this is not the reason for the existence of the church—the mission of Christ is to bring the presence of God to sinful and suffering humanity. A paradigm shift in the pastoral focus and pastoral practice is needed.

"Mi-Yittan,"[121] [OH] if Seventh-day Adventist pastors would equip themselves and their members in a trained ministry of healing to PLWHA, and would apply their knowledge and skill, combined with the expertise of medical practitioners in the local hospitals and medical facilities in communities, a far greater work for PLWHA will be accomplished. An effective, structured, well-managed, and well-functioning Home-Based Care program is needed wherever there is a Seventh-day Adventist presence that will make a difference in a ministry to PLWHA and their families.

> *"Every department of the local church should encourage and engage all members because a compassionate ministry of pastoral care to PLWHA is desperately needed."*

Every department of the local church should encourage and engage all members because a compassionate ministry of pastoral care to PLWHA is desperately needed. This ultimately is in line with the goal of the worldwide Seventh-day Adventist mission—to do the work of Jesus Christ on

---

[121] *"Mi-Yittan,"* Biblical Hebrew, like most languages, is sprinkled with idioms, words, or phrases that mean something different from what they immediately say. An example is *mi-yittan*, which is composed of two Hebrew words: *"mi,"* which is an interrogative *"who?"* and *"yittan,"* which means *"will give."* Thus, we have, *"Who will give?"* In Hebrew, this phrase expresses the idea of a wish or a desire of someone wanting something badly. For instance, in Psalm 14:7, David utters, *"Mi-yittan." "Oh, that the salvation of Israel were come out of Zion!"* The Hebrew doesn't say, *"Oh;"* it says *"Mi-Yittan."* See also Exodus 16:3; Job 6:8; Deuteronomy 5:29.

earth and to bring hope, healing, and deliverance to the sick and suffering both in the church and the communities! Christ's method alone can help us in a successful ministry of compassion. *"Mi-Yittan!"* [122]

2.11 Method: Jesus Christ's Method Alone Will Give True Success

The following principle given in the counsel from the Spirit of Prophecy (i.e. the writings of Ellen G. White) provides the Seventh-day Adventist Church with a secret to success in ministry and caring for the physical and spiritual needs of people, thus making sure that all barriers of prejudices are broken down, stigmatization is dealt with, and Christ is revealed:

> Christ's method alone will give true success in reaching the people. The Saviour mingled with men as one who desired their good. He showed His sympathy for them, ministered to their needs, and won their confidence. Then He bade them, "Follow Me."[123]

For more than a century the Seventh-day Adventist Church has taught Christ's method of reaching people and healing their diseases. These principles, implied in Christ's method above, are a guarantee for success in healing ministries. For decades around the world, these simple steps have saved many lives from illness and death. Jesus is our greatest example in touching lives in dignified ways and restoring their faith in Him who is the Life-giver. The Bible is clear that whenever Jesus passed through a village

---

[122] *[* 5. מִי with impf.:
    a) מִי יֹאמַר who may say … Jb 9:12;
    b) as an unreal wish (Brockelmann *Heb. Syn.* §9) מִי יְשִׂמֵנִי שֹׁפֵט 2S 15:4 Mal 1:10, Ju 9:29;
    • > מִי יִתֵּן as an optative particle Dt 28:67, with a following clause:
    • מִי יִתֵּן יָדַעְתִּי I wished I had known Jb 23:3, Nu 11:29;
Koehler, L., Baumgartner, W., Richardson, M. E. J., & Stamm, J. J. (1999). *The Hebrew and Aramaic Lexicon of the Old Testament* (electronic ed., p. 575). Leiden; New York: E.J. Brill.

[123] White, *The Ministry of Healing*, 143.

or town people were healed of their diseases and many more daily came for healing and deliverance from demon possession and evil spirits. The greater news from the Gospels is that after receiving the Master's touch, they became disciples of Christ.

Research and reports in Adventism throughout the years have been positive about the above secret of success, wherever these steps were followed:

The Saviour,

1. Mingled with people as One who desired their good;
2. He showed His sympathy for them;
3. He ministered to their needs;
4. He won their confidence and trust;
5. Then He invited them, "Follow Me."

True success in a ministry of healing can only be reached through giving study to Christ's method, and in South Africa the Seventh-day Adventist pastors and their congregations would do well to give study to the strengths and weaknesses in their current approaches to ministries to PLWHA. Many biblical examples throughout Jesus' ministry on earth as found in the New Testament are the evidences of the Word becoming "flesh, and dwelt among us"[124] and are the clear indications of fulfilment of the Old Testament prophetic foretelling of *"Immanuel,"*[125] God with us—Christ, coming to seek and to save the lost. "For God sent *not* His Son into the world *to condemn the world*; but that the world through him might be saved."[126] After the Saviour's ignominious death on the cross and His victorious resurrection, having been given all authority in heaven and earth, He gave the great commission to His eleven disheartened disciples, to "go and make disciples of all nations ... teaching them to obey

---

[124] John 1:14, KJV.
[125] Isaiah 7:14, NKJV; Matthew 1:23, NKJV.
[126] John 3:17, KJV.

everything I have commanded you."[127] At the same time, He gave them the assurance "I am with you always, to the very end of the age."[128] This great commission is ours today, to go into the whole world, but more specifically to the people of South Africa, and to bring the good news of the Gospel, healing, and deliverance from sin in the name of Jesus—This is the work of the church and the call to pastoral care. The great commission of our Lord was intended as an extension, a continuation of the presence God in the world, of *"Immanuel, God with Us,"* including to the PLWHA!

2.12 The Seventh-day Adventist Church: Current Policy on HIV and AIDS[129]

2.12.1 General Conference of Seventh-day Adventists' Official Statement on HIV and AIDS

The Seventh-day Adventist Church agrees that the HIV and AIDS epidemic is a devastating tragedy, and is spreading around the world, having already claimed millions of lives. The following discussion highlights the *Official Statement on HIV and AIDS* as issued by the General Conference, headquarters of the SDA Church:

> The Seventh-day Adventist Church recognizes that the HIV and AIDS epidemic is a serious problem decimating entire populations. In many countries of the world, it is taking many lives, including Seventh-day Adventist Church members.

---

[127] Matthew 28:19, 20, NIV.
[128] Matthew 28:20, NIV.
[129] https://1ref.us/t4 (accessed 5/6/2019): General Conference of the Seventh-day Adventist Church AAIM Official Statement on HIV-AIDS, with a selection from previous General Conference related statements. AAIM Board Meetings, October 2002 and April 2003. Reviewed in 2009. Reviewed June 2011.

The General Conference encourages that wherever there is a Seventh-day Adventist Church that the Adventist community be engaged in a ministry to PLWHA:

> In view of Jesus' Great Commission and example during His earthly ministry, as recorded in the Scriptures, The Seventh-day Adventist Church is involved in an active Ministry to fight this terrible disease, and to assist the infected and affected, through the work of all its Agencies, Departments, Churches, Educational and Medical Institutions.

The AAIM (Adventist Aids International Ministry) is a multi-departmental initiative, involving many ministries of the Church. Because of the shared mission and commission by Jesus Christ, a participation of all the Church's departments and agencies is encouraged.

It is true that HIV and AIDS related diseases affect every dimension of health: physical, mental, emotional, social, and spiritual. Also, stigmatization, rejection, isolation, employment denial, and segregation, produce increased abortion and suicide rates. Therefore, the Seventh-day Adventist Church recognizes their need to use scientifically proven, effective medical treatments and preventative measures. Their church leaders are all called upon to respond through initiatives in education, prevention, treatment, and community service.

> Just as Christ came to offer healing to a suffering world, so the Seventh-day Adventists are commissioned to compassionately care for those who suffer and are affected with HIV [and AIDS]. Church members can safely serve as caregivers, at home or in health care facilities, if they are educated in appropriate methods of doing so.[130]

---

[130] Ibid.

The Seventh-day Adventist Church advocates that "evidence overwhelmingly confirms the importance of building solid and positive relationships between married couples, parents and children, adults and youth, as the way to prevent 'at risk' behaviours."[131] Therefore, moral and spiritual support for the youth is encouraged from families and churches. The Church has also alerted its leaders and members through their statement on HIV and AIDS (2011) that public health research shows that there is a doorway of opportunity for education and prevention between the ages of five to fifteen years (for all children), before they become infected. In addition to education in the home by Adventist parents, the Seventh-day Adventist Church has departments such as the weekly Sabbath School, Pathfinders and Adventurers, Children's Ministries, as well the Family Ministries Department[132] that cater to educational skills, social skills, and life skills for this age group (five to fifteen years).

Young women fifteen to twenty-four years of age are more vulnerable than men to infection with the HI virus. Such information as communicated via the Department of Public Health should be used in the strategic planning of interventions of education and prevention. For this age group the Seventh-day Adventist Church's educational programs are to be implemented by the Adventist Youth Department, Ambassadors, Adventist Women's Ministries (AWM), and Young Adventist Women's Ministries (YAWM)[133] as well as Family Ministries and Sabbath School Departments, where young men and women can benefit by these programs as well as participate in initiatives for PLWHA and their affected families. In certain regions of the world, women at an early age suffer from strong sexual pressure. Empowerment of women and their training in negotiating skills to avoid sexual pressures could help decrease the number of infections.

> Less effort should be put forth in condemnation and more in education and redemptive approaches that seek to

---

[131] Ibid.
[132] Departments of the Seventh-day Adventist Church.
[133] Ibid.

allow each individual to be persuaded by the deep moving of the Holy Spirit.[134]

In addition to the above, The SDA Church gives special consideration and encouragement to the implementation of adequate sexual education in all SDA schools, colleges, and universities at all curricular levels, including Pathfinder Clubs. The Seventh-day Adventist curriculum framework called "God's Good Gift of Sexuality" could effectively be implemented to form the basis of sexual education from infancy to adulthood. This framework and all HIV and AIDS (and STIs) programs should be contextualized for relevant cultural and linguistic needs.

The following actions were taken by the worldwide Seventh-day Adventist Church:

2.12.2 Reference Documents

1. The General Conference of Seventh-day Adventists: *AIDS Statement*—1990.
2. *Birth Control*: A Seventh-day Adventist Statement of Consensus (256-99G)—Revised 9/14/99.
3. The following is a selection from the SDA "Statement on Meeting the Challenges of Sexually Transmitted Diseases" (161-98G) Revised 4/29/98.

2.12.3 Advances Have Been Made Along Several Lines

1. Research has provided more accurate data;
2. Benefits of using condoms to reduce unwanted pregnancy and the spread of STIs (included HIV-AIDS) have been documented;
3. Dangers of promiscuity have been recognized;

---

[134] https://1ref.us/t4 (accessed 5/6/2019).

4. More effective treatment has reduced the spread and progression of many STIs;
5. Risk of long-term emotional damage resulting from casual sex has been recognized; and
6. Support has grown for the position that abstinence from extramarital sex promotes sexual and emotional health.

It is of paramount importance to note that these advances above, despite their limitations, have proved beneficial and should be encouraged for their positive effects. Seventh-day Adventist caregivers should be encouraged to participate in promoting such efforts and deserve the support of church members as they do so. A pragmatic approach to dealing with these serious problems and challenges of and the use of appropriate interventions should by no means be interpreted as endorsement or encouragement of sexual activity outside marriage or of unfaithfulness within marriage. Instead, these efforts must be seen as compassionate attempts to prevent or reduce the negative consequences of illicit sexual behavior and sexual promiscuity. The Seventh-day Adventist Church places a high regard on the sanctity of the marriage relationship as a holy institution by God the Creator Himself.

> *"The Seventh-day Adventist Church places a high regard on the sanctity of the marriage relationship as a holy institution by God the Creator Himself."*

2.12.4 Official Statement of the Worldwide SDA Church on HIV and AIDS

At times, family members, and pastors, teachers, counsellors, physicians, and others in helping professions may find themselves working with individuals who, despite strong counsel, refuse to turn from sexual decadence and live by God's high standard of morality. In such cases, those entrusted with ministry may, as a last resort, counsel specific individuals to use contraceptive and prophylactic methods such as condoms in an attempt to prevent pregnancy and reduce the risk of spreading life-decimating STIs (included HIV-AIDS). Utmost care should be taken when making such an intervention to make it clear to the individual(s) and members of the community involved that this extreme measure should in no way be misconstrued as a scriptural sanction for sexual intimacy outside marriage. Such action on the part of professionals should be considered temporary and utilized only in individual cases. Though such interventions may provide a little time for grace to do its work in human hearts, they do not provide a viable long-term solution. The Church must remain committed to making the most of every opportunity to reinforce the wisdom of God's design for human sexuality and to calling men and women to the highest standard of moral conduct.

The *Seventh-day Adventist Church* affirms the biblical view of sexuality as a wholesome attribute of human nature created by God to be enjoyed and used responsibly in the sanctity of marriage as part of Christian discipleship.

The *Seventh-day Adventist Church* calls people to dedicate themselves before God to sexual abstinence outside the marriage covenant and sexual faithfulness to one's spouse. Apart from the wholesome expression of sexual intimacy in marriage, abstinence is the only safe and moral path for the Christian. In any other context, sexual activity is both harmful and immoral. This high standard represents God's intention for the use of His gift, and believers are called upon to uphold this ideal, regardless of the prevailing standards in the culture around them.

The *Seventh-day Adventist Church* recognizes the sinfulness of humanity. Human beings make mistakes, use poor judgment, and many deliberately choose to engage in sexual practices that are contrary to God's ideal. Others may know where to turn for help to live sexually pure lives. Nothing, however, can spare such individuals from the consequences of departing from the divine plan. Emotional and spiritual wounds left by sexual activity that violates God's plan inevitably leave scars. But the Church extends Christ's ministry of mercy and grace by offering God's forgiveness, healing, and restorative power. It must seek to provide the personal, spiritual, and emotional support that will enable the wounded to lay hold of the gospel's resources. The Church must also help persons and families identify and access the full network of professional resources available.

The *Seventh-day Adventist Church* recognizes as morally acceptable the use of contraceptive measures, including condoms, by married couples who seek to control conception. Condoms in particular may be indicated in some marital circumstances—for example, when one partner has been exposed to or has contracted a sexually transmitted disease, thus putting the spouse at high risk for infection.

On the other hand, the premarital or extramarital use of condoms—either in an attempt to lower the risk of unwanted pregnancy or to prevent the transmission of sexually transmitted diseases—raises moral concerns. These concerns must be considered in the context of the divine plan for human sexuality, the relationship between God's creative intent, and His regard for human frailty, the process of spiritual growth, and moral development within individuals, and the nature of the Seventh-day Adventist Church's mission.

Though condoms have proven to be somewhat effective in preventing pregnancy and the spread of disease, this does not make sex outside of marriage morally acceptable. Neither does this fact prevent the emotional damage that results from such behavior. The Church's appeal to youth and adults, believers and non-believers, is to live lives worthy of the grace extended to us in Christ, drawing as fully as possible upon divine and human resources to live according to God's ideal for sexuality.

The *Seventh-day Adventist Church* acknowledges that in cases where a married person may be at risk for transmitting or contracting a sexually transmitted disease such as Human Immunodeficiency Virus (HIV) from his or her marriage partner, the use of condom is not only morally acceptable but strongly recommended if the husband and wife decide to continue having sexual intercourse. Users of condoms must be alerted to the limits of their effectiveness in preventing the transmission of HIV infection and to the importance of using them properly.

2.12.5 An Appeal as Put Forth by the General Conference

The appeal as put forth by the General Conference of Seventh-day Adventists through AAIM is therefore as follows:

> We are facing the HIV and AIDS crisis that threatens the lives and well-being of many people, including church members. Both youth and adults are in peril. The Church must develop, without delay, a comprehensive strategy of education and prevention. The resources of health, social services, educational, ministerial, and other professionals, both within and without the Church, must be mobilized. This crisis demands priority attention—using every legitimate resource and method at the Church's disposal to target home, school, church, and community. The destiny of an entire generation of human beings is at stake, and we are in a race against time.[135]

1. See Birth Control: A Seventh-day Adventist Statement of Consensus (160-98G)
2. "Research indicates that condoms, when correctly used, have about a 97 percent success rate of prevention of pregnancy and about 85 to

---

[135] https://1ref.us/t4 (accessed 5/6/2019).

90 percent success rate in prevention of virus transmission, as used by the general population. In those groups who use them consistently and correctly, the effectiveness is about 97 percent."[136]

2.12.6 Conclusions on the General Conference Policy on HIV and AIDS

Main recommendations to fight STIs and HIV-AIDS: [137]
(2009 Update of the 1990 GC-AIDS Statement)

1. Promote education on sexuality according to biblical principles, and prevention on STIs and HIV-AIDS.
2. Uphold the ideal of abstinence from premarital sex.
3. Advocate premarital HIV testing for both potential partners as part of the church-based preparation for marriage.
4. Elevate God's ideal for faithfulness in marriage.
5. Encourage voluntary counselling and testing for understanding and early diagnosis on STIs, and HIV-AIDS.
6. Use of protective measures against sexually transmitted diseases, including HIV.
7. Compassionate care for those who suffer and are affected with HIV-AIDS.

2.13 The SAU (Southern Africa Union) of SDA Working Policy on HIV/AIDS[138]

2.13.1 Name and Territory of the Association

Name: The HIV/AIDS Ministries of the Southern Africa Union
Territory: Southern Africa Union (Lesotho, Namibia, South Africa, Swaziland)

---

[136] https://1ref.us/si (accessed 5/6/2019).
[137] https://1ref.us/sj (accessed 5/6/2019).
[138] HIV/AIDS Ministries, Southern Africa Union, "Working Policy on HIV/AIDS."

2.13.2 The Mission of the HIV and AIDS Ministries of the Southern Africa Union

To coordinate actions and resources to bring comfort, healing and hope to people infected and/or affected by HIV and AIDS, share a message of education and prevention to the **SAU** territory, and to accomplish what our Lord Jesus Christ has commissioned each of us to do.

2.13.3 The Vision of the SAU

1. To create "Centers of Hope and Healing" through our network of churches, medical, and educational institutions.
2. To mobilize our congregations through church-based support groups.
3. To bring practical solutions to those infected and affected by HIV and AIDS.
4. To apply the practical Gospel of Jesus Christ, church-by-church, person-by-person, and on a one-to-one basis.

2.13.4 The Purpose and Position Statement of the SAU of Seventh-day Adventists

The aim of the SAU policy above is to establish a clear framework within which the Southern Africa Union will:[139]

A. Manage the challenges and threats of HIV and AIDS to its employees at its Conferences, and Educational and Medical Institutions,
B. Provide guidelines for church leaders on how to relate and minister to PLWHA in their congregations and communities, create church-based support groups, and mobilize their congregations for a Ministry of Compassion,

---

[139] Ibid.

C. Endeavour to ensure that its members treat PLWHA in their employing organizations, churches and communities with Christian love and respect.

In South Africa[140] the increasing number of HIV infections rank highest in the world. It is a great cause for concern that the proportion of South Africans infected with HIV has increased from 10.6 percent in 2008 to 12.2 percent in 2012, according to the Human Sciences Research Council's (HSRC) National HIV Prevalence, Incidence and Behaviour Survey that was released in 2014. The total number of infected South Africans in 2014 stood at 6.4 million; 1.2 million more than in 2008.[141]

Among these figures of epidemic proportions in SAU territory are members of the Seventh-day Adventist Church living with HIV and AIDS. In spite of these good policies which the Seventh-day Adventist Church has in place, this recurring question remains: How can ministries to PLWHA be promoted and enhanced at a grassroots level? This research has found that it has become necessary to form an association for Seventh-day Adventist people living with HIV and AIDS.

2.14   The SAU-AAPLHA[142] Constitution

2.14.1   Name and Territory of the Association[143]:

1. The name of the group shall be: Association of Adventist People Living with HIV and AIDS (AAPLHA).
2. The territory served by the Association shall primarily be the area covered by the Southern Africa Union.

---

[140] The 2007 UNAIDS report estimated that 5,700,000 South Africans had HIV/AIDS, or just under **12 percent** of South Africa's population of 48 million. In the adult population the rate is 18.5 percent. The number of infected is larger than in any other single country in the world. HIV/AIDS in South Africa—Wikipedia, the free encyclopedia,
https://1ref.us/sk (accessed 5/6/2019).
[141] *Mail & Guardian* (April 1, 2014).
[142] AAPLHA: Association of Adventist People Living with HIV and AIDS.
[143] Article 1 of SAU-AAPLHA Constitution.

The SAU-AAPLHA Constitution is an eight-page document with clear stipulations and guidelines of name and territory, mission statement, vision, aims and objectives, membership of the association, management of the organization, duties of officers of management committee, an executive committee and their duties, meetings, finances, advisory board, and its by-laws.

2.14.2 Mission Statement of SAU-AAPLHA[144]

To provide an environment of dignity and respect with sustained life-affirming experience; and strengthen shared interests to improve quality of life for people living with HIV and AIDS.

2.14.3 Vision of SAU-AAPLHA[145]

1. To eradicate stigma and discrimination against people living with HIV and AIDS.
2. To increase awareness in the community so that PLWHA and those who are negative but are affected can work together towards zero new infections.
3. To create "Centers of Hope Healing" through network of churches, medical, and educational institutions.

2.14.4 Aims and Objectives of SAU-AAPLHA[146]

1. Community education and advocacy for the rights of PLWHA.
2. Counselling, support, and empowerment for those infected and affected.
3. Support special care programs for the orphans and vulnerable children due to HIV and AIDS.

---

[144] Article 2 of SAU-AAPLHA Constitution.
[145] Article 3 of SAU-AAPLHA Constitution.
[146] Article 4 of SAU-AAPLHA Constitution.

4. Vulnerability reduction through social, legal, and economic empowerment.
5. Promotion of voluntary counselling and testing, and status disclosure to encourage positive outlook and enjoy life-affirming experience.

2.15 The Adventist-AIDS International Ministry (AAIM)[147]

AAIM International has a Tri-Divisional Africa office located in Johannesburg, South Africa. This Adventist AIDS International office serves the territory of continental Africa and the Indian Ocean through the Adventist medical, educational, humanitarian, and religious institutions.

2.15.1 The AAIM Identity Statement

The AAIM is an international ministry of the Seventh-day Adventist Church that brings hope, love, and compassionate care and support to the people touched by the HIV and AIDS epidemic.

2.15.2 The AAIM Mission

> To coordinate actions and resources to bring comfort, healing and hope to people infected and/or affected by HIV/AIDS, share a message of education and prevention to the general population, and present a united front in order to accomplish what our Lord Jesus Christ has commissioned us to do.[148]

This mission statement of the AAIM ministries sums up the focus and objective of this book: an urgent call to the Seventh-day Adventist

---

[147] https://1ref.us/t4 (accessed 5/6/2019).
[148] Ibid.

Church in South Africa to coordinate, mobilize, and engage all its departments, institutions, and members in effective caring ministries to PLWHA through Home-Based Care.

2.15.3 The AAIM Vision

> We are creating "Centres of Hope and Healing" through our network of churches, medical and educational institutions, and church members. We are mobilizing our congregations through church based support groups. We are bringing practical solutions to those infected and affected by HIV and AIDS. We are applying the practical Gospel of Jesus Christ, field-by-field, church-by-church, and person-by-person, on a one to one basis. We are committed to the social responsibility of our church. We are helping to make HIV and AIDS history!

My personal appeal to the Seventh-day Adventist Church through this book is, *"Mi-Yittan," "Who will give?"* and *"Who will go?"* and work in God's field serving PLWHA and their families in our churches and in our communities in South Africa?

2.16 Ellen G. White and the Care of Orphans

A ministry to AIDS orphans is to be prioritized by the Seventh-day Adventist Church.

> Among all whose needs demand our interest, the widows and the fatherless have the strongest claims on our tender sympathy. They are the objects of the Lord's special care. They are lent to [Christian caregivers] in trust for God. "Pure religion and undefiled before God and the Father is this, to visit the fatherless and widows in their

affliction, and to keep himself unspotted from the world." James 1:27.[149]

The Seventh-day Adventist Church cannot afford to ignore or to rest on their laurels regarding the great need in the community for practical and creative ministries to AIDS orphans.

1. Ellen G. White left the Church with an abundance of guidance on the care and protection of orphans:

   > Many a father, who has died in the faith, resting upon the eternal promise of God, has left his loved ones in full trust that the Lord would care for them. And how does the Lord provide for these bereaved ones? He does not work a miracle in sending manna from heaven; He does not send ravens to bring them food; but He works a miracle upon human hearts, expelling selfishness from the soul and unsealing the fountains of benevolence. He tests the love of His professed followers by committing to their tender mercies the afflicted and bereaved ones.[150]

2. She also wrote extensively on pastoral care and a ministry of compassion and stressed the importance of the care of orphans. Serious counsel is given to "[l]et those who have the love of God open their hearts and homes to take in these children. It is not the best plan to care for the orphans in large institutions. If they have no relatives able to provide for them, the members of our churches should either adopt these little ones into their families or find suitable homes for them in other households."[151] "These children are in a special sense the ones whom Christ looks upon, whom it is an offense to Him to neglect. Every kind

---
[149] White, *Testimonies for the Church, Vol. 6*, 281.1.
[150] White, *Testimonies for the Church, Vol. 6*, 281.2.
[151] White, *Testimonies for the Church, Vol. 6*, 281.3.

act done to them in the name of Jesus is accepted by Him as done to Himself."[152]

3. It is a common occurrence that AIDS orphans are robbed of their property, grants, and their financial inheritance:

> Those who in any way rob them of the means they should have, those who regard their wants with indifference, will be dealt with by the Judge of all the earth 'Shall not God avenge His own elect, which cry day and night unto Him, though He bear long with them? I tell you that He will avenge them speedily.' 'He shall have judgment without mercy, that hath showed no mercy.' (Luke 18:7–8; 2:13)." God calls us to "'bring the poor that are cast out to our homes.' (Isaiah 58:7). Christianity must supply fathers and mothers and homes for these destitute ones. Compassion for the widow and orphan, manifested in prayers and corresponding deeds, will come up in remembrance before God, to be rewarded by and by.[153]

4. "The truth for this time embraces the whole gospel." A joint ministry is needed in pastoral care to PLWHA:

> Rightly presented [the joint efforts in ministry] will work in [all] the very changes that will make evident the power of God's grace on the heart[s] [of those we minister to]. It will do a complete work and develop a complete [person]." There ought to be no line "drawn between the genuine medical missionary work and the gospel ministry. Let these two blend in giving the invitation: 'Come; for all

---

[152] White, *Testimonies for the Church, Vol. 6*, 281.4.
[153] White, *Testimonies for the Church, Vol. 6*, 281.5.

things are now ready.' Let them be joined in an inseparable union, even as the arm is joined to the body.[154]

2.17 The Seventh-day Adventist Church and Health Ministries

Health ministries play a vital role as a major pillar within Seventh-day Adventist faith. The Church promotes teachings on health and healthful lifestyle practices as an essential part of Adventism and has a strong focus on healing ministries for its members and the members of the community. Seventh-day Adventists also view healing ministries as closely linked to gospel ministry:

> The Church believes its responsibility to make Christ known to the world includes a moral obligation to preserve human dignity by promoting optimal levels of physical, mental, and spiritual health.
>
> In addition to ministering to those who are ill, this responsibility extends to the prevention of disease through effective health education and leadership in promoting optimum health, free of tobacco, alcohol, other drugs, and unclean foods. Where possible, members shall be encouraged to follow a primarily vegetarian diet.[155]

2.18 Findings in Chapter Two

This chapter has extensively covered the history and the development of the Seventh-day Adventist Church in South Africa and presented a clear account of the value and advantages of a number of pillars of Adventist

---

[154] White, *Testimonies for the Church*, Vol. 6, 291.1.
[155] See Appendix #2: Departments in the Church for Ministry.

faith in ministries to PLWHA, which are to be taken into consideration in the incorporation of Home-Based Care into the pastoral ministry of the Seventh-day Adventist Church. These hallmarks within Adventism are much needed to equip, empower, and enable the larger Seventh-day Adventist Church community with a well-trained, skilled taskforce to provide an effective ministry of compassion and Christian care to PLWHA. The Seventh-day Adventist Church is also blessed with an army of skilled and professional church members who should engage in the training and equipping of its members as home-based caregivers, lay counsellors, home-school teachers, trainers in social skills, etc., so that the local congregations will become more involved in a structured Home-Based Care program.

These existing official policies on HIV and AIDS which the Seventh-day Adventist Church has in place should be communicated down from the SAU and Conference administration to the congregations and members at a grassroots level where active Home-Based Care ministries are to be organized in such a way that the local leaders and congregations take responsibility for their own members living with HIV and AIDS, particularly in poor communities.

> *"The Church promotes teachings on health and healthful lifestyle practices as an essential part of Adventism and has a strong focus on healing ministries for its members and the members of the community."*

The Seventh-day Adventist Church has members in the local congregations who are professional nurses, medical doctors, lawyers, physiotherapists, counsellors, psychologists, professors, lecturers, teachers, and pastors, as well as several other professions, such as businessmen, accountants, farmers, students, etc. Every possible profession and skill should be tapped into for volunteer service, in efforts to alleviate the plight of PLWHA in poor communities through practical and creative ministries. Even the youth and children can engage in creative friendship ministries to PLWHA and their families—children can minister to children and adults in various ways, such as visiting orphanages and sharing toys, reading Bible stories, etc. Retired church members are gems in a volunteer program to PLWHA. There is a work for each one to do. "No stone is to be left unturned" in attempts to curb the spread of HIV in the Seventh-day Adventist Church and the community and to care for the sick among us.

During my time of study at Stellenbosch University I had the privilege to gain practical experience as pastoral counsellor at clinics and Faith Based Organizations (FBO) in very poor communities and I have found that there is a definite link between poverty, HIV and AIDS, and the church. The experience as pastoral counsellor provided me with network connections and exposure to FBO's such as JL Zwane and the Presbyterian Church (to be discussed in chapter three), where these organizations ventured on Home-Based Care programs with great successes. Being passionate about pastoral care to terminally ill people, I have a burden to introduce such a ministry to the Seventh-day Adventist Church in South Africa where many members are suffering and dying of AIDS-related diseases in poorer communities.

The next chapter is a general investigation on how the HIV and AIDS epidemic challenges the traditional understanding of "church" as an institution; how other faith-based groups are managing these challenges; and how they can help the Seventh-day Adventist Church formulate their own Home-Based Care programs using their existing resources.

CHAPTER THREE

The HIV and AIDS Epidemic as Challenge to Other Ecclesiologies: Towards an Eclectic Contextual Home-Based Care in the SDA Church

This chapter is a general investigation on how the HIV and AIDS epidemic in South Africa challenges traditional understandings of the church as an institution. Study will be given to hierarchical and clerical models with the emphasis on the role of clergy—pastoral care to PLWHA involves a ministry of compassion that is willing to bring the presence of God to the sick and suffering persons in need of comfort and care. In chapter two my research revealed that at the administrative level, that is, General Conference, Union, and Conference level, the Seventh-day Adventist Church has good policies in place to cater to the needs of PLWHA. Though, as pointed out in Chapter 1.3, the findings also raise concerns that the pastor to member ratio (averaging 1:554) makes it impossible for the pastor alone to carry the responsibility of caring for PLWHA. This chapter will give study to examples of existing ecclesiologies[156] who have successfully managed to offer community-based care that focuses on "being there" where the PLWHA are, as a guide for Seventh-day Adventists to develop their own Home-Based Care projects at a grassroots level as opposed

---

[156] The term "ecclesiology" refers to the branch of theology that is concerned with the nature and function of the church in fulfilling its mission.

to its traditional hierarchical and clerical approaches to pastoral care in the past.

3.1 HIV and AIDS: A Social Malady in South African Society

We live in a society where the social maladies of human existence are inescapable. The scourge of the ever increasing, daily escalating numbers of HIV infections in South Africa is a reality of this generation. HIV and AIDS are part and parcel of twenty-first century existence throughout the world, and South Africa is faced with the reality of being the country with the highest rate of HIV infections and the subsequent AIDS-related deaths in the world. Along with these alarming facts are the ever-increasing figures of AIDS orphans and child-headed homes where both parents have died of AIDS-related diseases. The sad reality of the South African situation is that most PLWHA are among the poorest communities in the country. HIV and AIDS and poverty are twins that walk hand in hand until death comes for the victims of an HIV infection.

The truth about the conversation on the topic of HIV and AIDS is that this infectious disease is a human condition, which to date has been categorized as an incurable infectious disease—and is therefore an ongoing dialogue for the stakeholders of HIV and AIDS management, care, and counselling. HIV and AIDS has reached epidemic proportions in many countries around the world and in South Africa this is no exception. While it is true that HIV and AIDS affect some communities more adversely than others, this is a topic which we cannot ignore. Because HIV and AIDS is a widespread reality for the South African society, every citizen should live in awareness of the far-reaching effects of the disease and regard themselves as stakeholders of a campaign against HIV infection.

3.2 Five Imperative Questions Forcing Us to Come to the Party of Stakeholders of HIV and AIDS: From a Hierarchical and Clerical Structure to a Grassroots Ecclesiology

The following five imperative questions force us to join the party of stakeholders of the HIV and AIDS epidemic and are useful in a paradigm shift from a hierarchical and clerical structure to a grassroots ecclesiology:

1. How has HIV and AIDS affected the community where I live?
2. How has HIV and AIDS affected the faith community where I worship?
3. How can those from faith communities join resources—materially, spiritually, and financially—and offer help and healing, intervention, and relief to PLWHA, and in the process become more effective faith-based communities themselves?
4. How does the faith community where I serve respond to the HIV and AIDS epidemic, and do they have an existing ministry of compassion and care for PLWHA?
5. How has my church provided and facilitated training and education programs to equip and empower its members for a ministry of compassion in Home-Based Care to PLWHA?

To further encourage the dialogue on the Church's response to the HIV and AIDS epidemic and the urgently needed intervention, I have embarked on a general investigation on how the HIV and AIDS epidemic challenges traditional understandings of the Church as an institution, and the role of clergy. Pastoral care to PLWHA involves a ministry of compassion that is willing to bring healing and the presence of God to the sick and suffering persons in need of comfort and care.

The HIV and AIDS epidemic has challenged people's perceptions and basic understanding of what it means to be "church" and it has particularly brought the traditional clerical paradigm under the spotlight.

The epidemic has raised the intriguing question: "How has the Church responded to the needs of PLWHA?" The Seventh-day Adventist Church has need of establishing Home-Based Care programs and projects as a way forward in caring for their members living with HIV and AIDS. Since the first occurrences of HIV and AIDS in South Africa, Christian churches have run Home-Based Care programs, which catered effectively to the multiplicity of needs of PLWHA. I have, however, since 1998, been involved in pastoral care and counselling as well as Home-Based Care to terminally ill people, including PLWHA, and am confident that given the right direction, guidance, and "tools," the Seventh-day Adventist Church in South Africa can make a significant contribution to the lives of PLWHA. Among its members are people living with HIV and AIDS. Many PLWHA have turned to the Seventh-day Adventist Church for help and have joined the Church. For an understanding of Home-Based Care, we will look at some examples that can help the Seventh-day Adventist Church to develop their own HBC program.

For a practical and effective ecclesiological approach to a compassionate ministry of care to PLWHA, the Church as a whole and as the body of Christ should get on board in joint multi-dimensional ministries which cater to the multiplicity of needs of HIV and AIDS sufferers. Several theological indicators are of paramount importance in an effective ministry:

- **Koinonia:** The Church as the body of Christ ought to function as "a practical and effective conduit of God's love and compassion to the poor and HIV and AIDS sufferers, it should translate/concretise the gospel to real-life situations. The concretisation could be possible through the mutual care of the *koinonia*. In order to do this, an ecclesial model should shift from a stance of apathy towards one of empathy and contextual engagement."[157]
- **Diakonia:** This is a Christian theological term from Greek that encompasses the call to serve the poor and oppressed. This should then

---

[157] Magezi (2005), 77.

include every member of the family of God to display a willingness to engage in service for others. This calls for a systems approach to pastoral care. "The church becomes a horizon where the Word (theory or reflection) and action or praxis merge, i.e. the mutual care and service (*diakonia*) within the fellowship of the body (church)."[158]
- **Leitourgia:** Refers to a form according to which public religious worship, especially Christian worship, is conducted. Christian worship should be inclusive if it is to be a true representation and reflection of the body of Christ or family of God metaphors. A Christian community of faith will therefore ensure that all worshipers, including PLWHA, are welcome to participate in all services of the church.
- **Kerygma:** Similarly, kerygma, which refers to the preaching or proclamation of the Christian gospel, will be an inclusive message of hope and healing to all worshipers and members of the body of Christ.

In order for a practical ministry to be inclusive it will pay attention to the theological indicators above for a holistic approach to a compassionate Home-Based Care ministry.

Moetlo, Pengpid, and Peltzer state:[159]:

> [1] Home-based care refers to the provision of health services by formal and informal caregivers within the home. The aim of home-based care is ultimately to "promote, restore and maintain a person's maximum level of comfort, function and health, including care towards a dignified death." [2] The WHO [1] foresees home-based care as an integral and integrated aspect of health care. Home-based care is defined as the care that the health consumer (beneficiary) can "access nearest to home, which engages

---

[158] Ibid.

[159] Moetlo, Pengpid & Peltzer, 2011, An Evaluation of the Implementation of Integrated Community Home-Based Care Services in Vhembe District, South Africa, *Indian Journal of Palliative Care*, vol. 17, no 2, May–Aug 2011. Available from https://1ref.us/sl (accessed 5/6/2019).

participation by people, responds to the needs of people, encourages traditional community lifestyle and creates responsibilities."

In his epic *Cura Vitae*, Prof. Louw helps us in our understanding of an ecclesiological approach:

> The church is a strategically located and recognised institution. As a credible institution, it networks and mobilises resources from agencies, while at the same time being closely linked to the community. The local church can function as a crucial resource, channel and link to the community, thereby addressing the needs of the poor people. And through designing a congregational home-based pastoral care ministry, the congregation can reach out and provide support to affected people. In so doing, the church does not only perform a social function to the HIV-affected and poor families, but acts in accordance with the calling of mediating God's kingdom.[160]

Prof. Louw's view above provides us with a good point of departure for the establishment of Home-Based Care from an ecclesial Christian spiritual perspective. In order to provide successful and effective care to PLWHA in South Africa I agree with Prof. Louw that "for this approach the communal concept of African people *umunthu ungumunthu ngabathu* (a person is a person because of other people/or a person is a person through other persons), commonly called *Ubuntu*, is instrumental and an invaluable building block" in a ministry of pastoral care.

The Seventh-day Adventist Church would do well to embrace a ministry of care to the poor in the community and to show interest in the needs of PLWHA. Seventh-day Adventists are known to be warm people and

---

[160] Louw (2008), 452.

welcoming to strangers and visitors, and a Home-Based Care program will provide them with golden opportunities to truly be the currency of heaven through the gracious service of love to the vulnerable victims of HIV and AIDS. Disinterested benevolence and acts of kindness will most probably introduce scores to the heart of God when they experience the Christian love of the Seventh-day Adventists. The disadvantaged poor of South Africa need to feel the loving embrace and mercy of God, and Seventh-day Adventists are able to extend these to PLWHA through Home-Based Care ministries—the age-old home visitation programs should be revived as its members enter the homes of the sick and care for them.

While the Seventh-day Adventist Church for years already has had good policies on HIV and AIDS in place, the Church should become more actively involved at the local level and get on board in helping to lighten the burden of an HIV and AIDS epidemic in South Africa. There are several other existing faith communities and Faith Based Organizations (FBOs) who for decades already have successful Home-Based Care programs where care is being provided to PLWHA in the comfort of their own home by their family, friends, relatives, the church, and their community in a dignified and loving manner, even until their dying moments.

> *"The disadvantaged poor of South Africa need to feel the loving embrace and mercy of God, and Seventh-day Adventists are able to extend these to PLWHA through Home-Based Care ministries."*

The following are reasons worthy for the introduction and the establishment of good Home-Based Care initiatives and programs run by Seventh-day Adventists:

1. For an effective HBC program, an ecclesiology of community-based care focuses on bringing the presence of God, as the Great Physician, into the homes of the sick person. Healing can only take place when the sick person encounters the merciful touch of Omnipotence.

2. Due to the connection with HIV and AIDS and poverty in rural areas, there is a need for local support systems. Communities of faith are often the only reliable support system in townships/locations where the poor live. In every community, ecclesial structures are already in place and there is a Seventh-day Adventist Church in most of our communities.
3. Due to the connection between the church and the homes of members living with HIV and AIDS, the Church has the "right" to enter the homes to offer care.
4. Through the connection between the pastoral paradigm, e.g., the shepherding perspective, and the call of God to care for the lost, vulnerable, injured, and hurting lambs belonging to the flock, pastoral care moves to where the PLWHA are.
5. The conception and connection of *koinonia* thus will draw the pastoral attention to the suffering, helplessness, and vulnerability of PLWHA, thereby motivating the pastor and the church to create and maintain good support systems for PLWHA.
6. The connection of *diakonia* and outreach puts the Church at the forefront to meet the needs of PLWHA, irrespective of their religion, race, culture, lifestyle, orientation, or gender.

Since 1998 I have done extensive training in the field of HIV and AIDS and palliative care, and have gained clinical experience as a Clinical Pastoral Counsellor, which included Home-Based Care, at the following three treatment centers for PLWHA:

1. **Helderberg Hospice[161], Somerset West**—during 1998–2001 I was assigned to the Helderberg Hospice for my practical credit hour requirements for undergraduate degree in BA theology pastoral ministry program, which extended into volunteer basis service at the hospice. At the time, the hospice was a sixteen-bed in-patient NGO facility

---

[161] https://1ref.us/sm (accessed 5/6/2019).

offering palliative care service to the terminally ill patients from the Helderberg basin, Somerset West, South Africa. It was required of me to fulfil duties like pastoral care and counselling; Home-Based Care; Grief counselling to bereaved families of (for) both in/out-patients. The hospice also sent me on further advanced training courses in pastoral care. This experience proved to be rewarding, enriching, and empowering, and it also gave me a sense of vision for a similar ministry for the Seventh-day Adventist Church. Many patients and families were blessed by this ministry and many testimonies were recorded where patients and families responded positively to pastoral care. The Seventh-day Adventist Church indeed has a role to play and a moral obligation towards PLWHA.

2. **Ikhwezi Day Hospital and Clinic** is located in Nomzamo, Cape Town and is a government/public organization and a day hospital offering primary health care to the Lwandle and Nimzamo communities. The hospital has an excellent HIV, AIDS, and TB-related treatment center offering care, counselling, and support services to PLWHA. I was assigned to this hospital during 2007 where I completed my practical clinical work.

    Ikhwezi Clinic is a community-oriented, primary health care organization and their program monitors its patients closely and effectively, and proactively assists them to work towards improved health. The clinic has strong empowerment programs and shows great interest in the well-being of families in their community. They are an accredited antiretroviral (ARV) treatment initiation and on-going treatment site. There I was assigned to work alongside the medical doctor and the nursing staff as well as with the home-based caregivers, who all worked together well as a networking team having the patients' best interest at heart. When necessary, Ikhwezi refers patients to Tygerberg Hospital for additional care and treatment. Ikhwezi distributes fortified porridge and nutritional milkshakes to underweight patients as well as malnourished TB and HIV patients. Every month the hospital runs a support group for HIV-positive people.

3. **JL Zwane[162] Community Centre, in Gugulethu, Cape Town, South Africa.** I chose to do an in-depth study on the JL Zwane model of Home-Based Care—this FBO provides sterling services to their members of the Presbyterian Church as well as for the members of the community. This is a model that I would like to propose as a viable model for the Seventh-day Adventist Church to consider in their formulation of a CHBC program.

3.3 The JL Zwane Memorial Church, Gugulethu, Cape Town, Responds to HIV and AIDS

JL Zwane is a Faith Based Organization (FBO) established by the JL Zwane Memorial Presbyterian Church, offering intervention and care to its church members, as well as members of the community, living with HIV and AIDS.

Nobis Xapile states that:

> Gugulethu is one of the areas in the Western Cape where people have really suffered the negative consequences of migratory labour system. Because of the migratory labour system the family structure was completely destroyed. Many children that grow up in black townships have no idea what family life is. As a result they do not value relationships let alone marriage. The minister in the above congregation says ever since he started his ministry there, in 1989, he has married only 13 couples but has baptized more than 1000 children. People cannot commit to marriage because they cannot relate to it.[163]

---

[162] https://1ref.us/sn (accessed 5/6/2019).

[163] Xapile, N. 2005. "The Faith Based Organization Response to HIV/AIDS: A Case Study of the JL Zwane Memorial Church in Gugulethu, Cape Town." MPhil (HIV Management), University of Stellenbosch.

The security of the family structure plays a vital role in fighting the rapid spread of HIV. In a community such as the one described above with no family structure and/or lacking a strong family value system, HIV thrives. Children practice what they observe in adults when they themselves grow up. The disadvantages of growing up in such communities often become the challenges that the church and the pastor face—it usually automatically becomes the role and responsibility of the church to act as extended family for its members.

Most cities and towns in South Africa will have at least one or more poor, densely-packed-into-one-area, overpopulated township or *"location"*[164] as most people call it, which is a poverty-stricken area with poor access for maintenance, electricity, water, and sanitation. In most cases people who live there have migrated to cities and towns from other poverty-stricken areas to be closer to ARV treatment and have better job opportunities. Also, it is very common in locations like these that people turn to the church for relief, help, intervention, and survival. In many instances there are no schools, but inevitably there will be a church.

It is against this kind of backdrop, in 1996, that JL Zwane Memorial Church took action and became a sanctuary and a place of refuge for its members. Members of the congregation were dying and, in many instances, more than one person from the same family would be HIV-positive and/or have advanced (Stage 4) AIDS.

Xapile cited:

> For an example one family had three sisters who were HIV positive and they developed full-blown AIDS at the same time. They died one after another, leaving seven children with no one to look after them. The church was

---

[164] In South Africa, the terms *township, location*, or *khasi* are commonly used for an overpopulated, underdeveloped, urban living area.

then faced with the responsibility of raising and supporting these children.[165]

The HIV and AIDS epidemic wreaks havoc in congregations, especially in poverty-stricken areas. For a number of years, I have heard the complaints from fellow Seventh-day Adventist pastors working in townships. The challenges, demands, and needs of PLWHA and their families are overwhelming, taxing, burdensome, and draining. Most pastors in the Seventh-day Adventist Church are assigned to large districts, with the number congregations in their care for which they are responsible ranging from no less than six and up to twelve or more congregations. The high frequency of AIDS-related deaths and funerals can become stressful and draining. Funerals far exceed the number of weddings and the figures of orphans are ever increasing.

While HIV and AIDS remain rife in several cultural communities, talking about it there is taboo, which increases the difficulty of changing the status quo. Stigmatization and rejection, and even the threat being disowned by their families, are among the greatest fears of PLWHA. Members of the Seventh-day Adventist Church do not talk about this huge problem of HIV and AIDS that is ravaging the church and the community. Certain cultures and communities, including faith communities, do not allow or encourage open talk and discussions on the issue of sexuality and HIV and AIDS. This means that there is a great need for awareness, training and education, care and support to bring treatment and intervention programs closer to the PLWHA.

After embarking on a situational analysis and needs assessment of the JL Zwane Memorial Presbyterian Church and the community, they started a model FBO in ministry to PLWHA that included a strong Home-Based Care program.

---

[165] Xapile, N. 2005. "The Faith Based Organization Response to HIV/AIDS: A Case Study of the JL Zwane Memorial Church in Gugulethu, Cape Town." MPhil (HIV Management), University of Stellenbosch.

3.3.1 The JL Zwane Mission Statement[166]

To lessen the suffering brought about by the HIV and AIDS epidemic, by being dedicated to providing care and support to people living with and affected by HIV and AIDS.

3.3.2 The JL Zwane Aims[167]

- To live out what God requires of us as a church in the face of HIV and AIDS.
- To eliminate the stigma and discrimination brought about by HIV and AIDS.
- To provide care and support to people living with and affected by HIV and AIDS.
- To address the nutritional needs.
- To break the silence surrounding HIV and AIDS at the same time giving a face to the epidemic.
- To educate members of the community about HIV and AIDS.
- To find ways of combating the spread of HIV.

In my experience at JL Zwane, the pastor, staff, and volunteers were all committed and dedicated in service to PLWHA to achieve the above mission statement and aims. The JL Zwane ministry team, who are themselves PLWHA, would also gladly tour throughout the country to do fundraising concerts, as well as train and empower other FBOs and churches on such tours.

---

[166] Xapile (2005), 7.
[167] Ibid.

3.3.3 The JL Zwane Home-Based Care Program

According to Xapile, the Home-Based Care program arose from the need of PLWHA attending their church for care because hospitals in the area could not cope with the increasing numbers of people in the community who were sick. The support group facilitators, who were employees at the local community clinics, were also the initial volunteers to do Home-Based Care. This was quite stressful on the volunteers, as they did this after working hours. However, there were advantages in that these facilitators found it easy to refer patients to the local doctors, "as a relationship already existed between the church and the local clinics."[168]

Initially the people's ignorance regarding Home-Based Care was a problem. Also, they had no concept of volunteering. The help of St. Luke's Hospice staff was called in to educate the community and to train volunteers. Funding such an HBC program was another challenge. In 2002 JL Zwane received a donation specifically for their Home-Based Care program, and partnerships were formed with St. Luke's Hospice. Today the JL Zwane/St. Luke's Hospice is situated on the church premises with a qualified social worker and professional nursing staff who run it. Many volunteers receive training in HBC and become paid employees of the church.[169]

Xapile states:

> This is a much-needed service in our community considering the number of people living with HIV/AIDS...Our strength should be in prevention strategies, trying to combat the spread of HIV but until then Home-Based care is very important [sic].[170]

---

[168] Xapile (2005), 10.
[169] Xapile (2005), 11.
[170] Ibid.

Next, we will look at an Afro-Christian ministry to PLWHA as another example of an ecclesiology engaging in Home-Based Care, in an attempt to investigate their approaches to HBC.

3.4 An Afro-Christian Ministry to People Living with HIV and AIDS in South Africa[171]

Matsobane J. Manala, from the Department Practical Theology at the University of South Africa, in an academic article wrote on "An Afro-Christian Ministry" to people living with HIV/AIDS in South Africa asserts:

> In order for the church to play a relevant and meaningful role in combating the HIV/Aids epidemic, it is necessary that the church should be informed of the existential situation of persons living with HIV/Aids. This information is vital for raising awareness and engendering sensitivity among Christians. In the context of such awareness of and sensitivity to human pain and suffering, the community of the faithful should be moved to heed Christ's call to show neighbourly love. The possible role of the church in caring for those who are already infected with HIV is defined.[172]

Matsobane Manala believes that the HIV and AIDS epidemic "is cause for great frustration to the developing countries in their attempts to improve the quality of life of their citizens." Furthermore, he states that "HIV/Aids in South Africa demands a specific approach to the Christian ministry in which the African world-view is acknowledged."[173] In order to run a successful contextual Home-Based Care program, it is therefore of utmost importance that pastors and all who will engage in ministry to

---

[171] https://1ref.us/so (accessed 5/6/2019).
[172] Manala (2005).
[173] Ibid.

PLWHA are adequately informed on paradigms within the African spirituality, tradition, and culture.

The HIV and AIDS epidemic undoubtedly is one of the fiercest challenges ever facing Christian communities worldwide, and particularly in South Africa. Dreyer, as cited by Manala, states in this regard: "I would like to argue that in the continuing struggle for justice in South Africa, HIV/Aids presents an important challenge for theology in general and for practical theology in particular." Christian ministry and pastoral care focus on services to the church members and the community that are concerned with proclaiming the gospel of Jesus Christ and truths about the kingdom of God.

> "The HIV and AIDS epidemic undoubtedly is one of the fiercest challenges ever facing Christian communities worldwide, and particularly in South Africa."

> These services include imparting Christian ethical and moral values and conduct, as well as offering prayers for those who are in need. These services should emanate from and be founded upon the unconditional love and acceptance of Christians as ambassadors for Christ.[174]

In an attempt to highlight the value of an Afro-Christian approach, Manala draws the attention of Christian ministers and communities of faith to the importance being cognizant of African spirituality and the existential experiences and expectations of PLWHA.

The Afro-Christian approach takes seriously the existential and pastoral realities relating to people living with HIV and AIDS and seeks to integrate those values from the African and the Christian traditions that are meaningful and life-giving in service of the weak and marginalized people. It considers the African worldview as the basis for the Christian

---

[174] Ibid.

ministry to people of Africa in their experiential needs. The notion of "Afro-Christian" suggests that the Christian ministry in Africa should be genuinely African and Christian. Manala sees great potential for dynamic and efficient caring in the Christian ministry that is constructed on a two-fold foundation of Biblical and African cultural values.[175]

3.4.1 Contextual Aspects in the Afro-Christian Approach

The following contextual aspects are highlighted in the Afro-Christian approach:

1. "[Local] culture [is] the primary factor in the method of doing African theology and spirituality. At the moment the teaching method is of Western orientation and engages African experience as an afterthought.[176]
2. A Christian ministry that is constructed on a two-fold foundation of biblical and African cultural values. [177]
3. A ministry that encompasses the Ubuntu[178] philosophy, which is the predominant context of Biblical narratives, based on the four pillars of:
    i. Community (*koinonia*) both vertical and horizontal,
    ii. Mutuality,
    iii. Self-sacrifice for the sake of the other, and
    iv. The belief in God's healing power can be observed in these two communities.

---

[175] Ibid.

[176] Seoka (1997), 1.

[177] The biblical story about the life and work of the early Christian church as narrated in Acts 2:43–47 reveals the lifestyle that is characterised by close kinship, mutuality, self-sacrifice for the sake of the other, and prayerfulness. This lifestyle and the values of the Christian community reminds one of the African Ubuntu lifestyle. Four important pillars, namely community (koinonia) both vertical and horizontal, mutuality, self-sacrifice for the sake of the other, and the belief in God's healing power can be observed in these two communities. African people are known for their love of and concrete commitment to community. They are indeed a mutual community (Shorter, 1978, 27).

[178] The African way of life in which people believe that they are, because others are, and in which they believe, work for, and live in mutuality and interdependence.

4. Another characteristic that the African community shares with the Christian community is their belief in the God of love and in mutual love.

In order for any Christian ministry to be successful it is vital that study and consideration be given to the cultural context. The Afro-Christian approach emphasizes the culture of the people whom the gospel and Christianity reach, thus making culture the primary factor in the method of doing African theology and spirituality.

3.4.2   The Afro-Christian Approach, Ubuntu, and Patriarchy

As much as Manala values the philosophy and benefits of Ubuntu, he hastens to stress that the Afro-Christian approach is flawed and that he is opposed to the negative effects of a ministry of compassion which engenders patriarchy, and therefore highlights the following negative aspects of Afro-Christian tradition:

> Patriarchy is a destructive powerhouse and a serious problem. African societies, in spite of the enviable Ubuntu philosophy, are deeply patriarchal. The problem inherent in patriarchal societies is that they are gender-insensitive and oppressive to women, a situation that predisposes, precipitates and perpetuates HIV infection. Men make all the sex-related decisions which women as "minors" have no right to oppose, however unfair and unsafe these decisions may be.[179]

The evils of patriarchy can best be grasped when one carefully heeds the words of Nyambura Njoroge:[180]

---

[179] https://1ref.us/so (accessed 5/6/2019).
[180] Njoroge, N. "The Missing Voices: African Women Doing Theology." *Journal of Theology for Southern Africa* (1997), 99, 77–83. As quoted in Manala.

Patriarchy is a destructive powerhouse, with systematic and normative inequalities as its hallmark. It also affects the rest of the creation order. Its roots are well entrenched in society as well as the church—which means we need well-equipped and committed women and men to bring patriarchy to its knees.

Knowledge is power. It is therefore the duty of the ministers to sensitize their healing communities to the contextual needs of PLWHA and to empower its members for a ministry of greater compassion and meaningful action that is *Sola Scriptura* and carries the hallmarks and merits of the gospel of Jesus Christ. The Afro-Christian approach is valuable in an attempt to transform any Christian ministry into a dynamic endeavor of service to PLWHA, however, I would agree with Manala and challenge the deeply entrenched, adverse effects of a patriarchal system on women, who are among the vast majority of PLWHA.

> "Knowledge is power. It is therefore the duty of the ministers to sensitize their healing communities to the contextual needs of PLWHA and to empower its members for a ministry of greater compassion and meaningful action."

Manala further argues the question on whether to advocate embracing the proposed Afro-Christian approach:

> I however do not think that patriarchy should be allowed to jeopardise opportunities for the design of a potentially helpful in Afro-Christian ministry to PLWHA, the approach should, as Ackermann (1993:21) so eloquently states, embody the ethical demands of the reign of God, namely justice, love, freedom and shalom. African theology within which the proposed Afro-Christian approach resides, therefore needs to purge itself of the evils of

sexism. In other words, it ought to reread and reinterpret the biblical texts that are life-denying to women. Masenya (2005:194) suggests that the present androcentric biblical hermeneutics should be challenged. The suggested biblical hermeneutics should acknowledge the woman as a human person in her own right, not as an attachment to a male partner. The suggestion therefore places the respect and honour of women at the centre of our theologising, if it is to contribute positively towards the Christian ministry to people living with HIV/Aids in Africa. Only then will the proposed Afro-Christian ministry to people living with HIV/Aids be acceptable, especially to women.[181]

The Catholic Church as a community of faith has been an outstanding source of relief work for decades, and especially so since the arrival of HIV and AIDS in South Africa. It has well-structured and established HIV centers throughout the country. We can learn much from the tireless humanitarian work done by the Catholic Church, for all churches face the same challenges in their ministry to PLWHA in South Africa. We will examine their experience in HIV and AIDS, seeking insights into some of the common challenges in a ministry to PLWHA.

3.5 The Catholic Church in Rural South Africa and HIV and AIDS

3.5.1 The Church and AIDS in South Africa Thirty Years After the Discovery of HIV

I have chosen to include the work of the Catholic Church as a final investigation on denominational responses to HIV and AIDS in South Africa. In my observation the Catholic Church has for years already been actively engaged

---

[181] Manala (2005).

in relief work and intervention to PLWHA. In many instances initiatives of the Catholic Church have surpassed those of the local government.

The following report and investigation are taken from a 20 January 2013 Vatican Radio interview conducted by Vatican News.[182]

3.5.1.1 The Catholic Church Responds to Pertinent Questions

1. How has the Catholic Church responded to the AIDS epidemic in Southern Africa since the discovery of the HIV virus thirty years ago?
2. How has the scenario changed in a nation where well over 5 million people are living with HIV and AIDS—the highest number of infected people in any country?
3. What are the prospects and the challenges?
4. What about the Church's role in caring for the sick and the orphaned?

These above were only a few of the questions on the issues pertinent to the scourge of an HIV and AIDS epidemic addressed and analyzed at a conference entitled "Catholic Responses to AIDS in Southern Africa, 30 Years After the Discovery of HIV." The conference took place from Sunday 20th to Tuesday 22nd January 2013 at St. Joseph's Theological Institute in the South African Kwa-Zulu Natal region.

Several participants at the Conference were Cardinal Wilfred Napier, Fr. Michael Czerny, Sr. Alison Munro, Bishop Kevin Dowling, and others who have been in the front line in the battle against HIV and AIDS and in caring for the victims for many, many years. The Vatican Radio's spokesperson, Linda Bordoni, conducted an interview with Bishop Kevin Dowling, who is the bishop of Rustenberg, South Africa. Dowling had been approached specifically to address the conference on the "Catholic Responses to HIV and AIDS in the rural local church" setting.

Bishop Kevin Dowling, who is the founder of the "Tapologo HIV/AIDS Project and Hospice" in Rustenberg, has been witnessing the

---

[182] https://1ref.us/sp (accessed 5/6/2019).

ravaging scars of the HIV and AIDS epidemic in South Africa close-up, and how it wiped out many infected and affected since his appointment to the Diocese of Rustenberg in 1991.

Rustenberg is a predominantly rural mining community, where the platinum mines are situated. Over the years, Rustenberg has attracted masses of migrant workers from even poorer rural areas in South Africa. The mine companies have also over the years recruited mine workers from other neighboring countries.

According to Bishop Dowling:

> So you have mine workers housed in hostels and huge migration of many people, particularly destitute women from rural areas. These people, he explains, set up homes in shacks of zinc and wood, in terrible conditions. They are all illegal so there are no services provided. This results in a lethal combination of extreme poverty, desperate people and mine workers who have left their homes to work away on the mines for many months. Thus the HIV infection rate, as a result of the socio-economic culture effect, is very high in the area and it is increasing.[183]

Given this harsh back drop of the spread of the HIV and AIDS epidemic, Bishop Dowling says the realization of the consequences of this reality is what drove him to start the Tapologo project.

The Rustenburg HIV and AIDS project is a very good example of a typical, poverty-stricken rural area that is a breeding ground for a fast-spreading epidemic:

- The link between poverty and the HIV and AIDS disease;
- The ever-increasing number of impoverished women who live in the illegal shack settlements around the mines;

---

[183] https://1ref.us/sp (accessed 5/6/2019).

- The increasing number of women who are forced into prostitution to feed themselves and their children;
- "Survival sex": Becoming the only means women and young girls have of surviving, they engage in unprotected sex for money with men who have the money, and they are the men who are employed at the mines or are contract workers and who have jobs;
- Absence of proper family system: It is common in urban and rural areas that men who have left their families behind in other countries or in rural areas and spend months alone in the hostels, engage in sexual relationships with multiple partners.

The "combination of desperate women, men who have money but who don't have their wives with them is the socio-economic cultural reality," Bishop Dowling says, "that is responsible for the dangerous lifestyle of these women who just want to survive."

Bishop Dowling raises the point of the uniqueness of the South African situation, which is of utmost importance to this subject:[184]

1. That "the first 10 to 15 years from the discovery of the virus were lost to our response as a country because we were totally engaged in the horrendous struggle against apartheid."
2. From the 1980s when former President Nelson Mandela was released, until the democracy in 1994, everything was focused on the struggle for democracy.
3. The HIV infections and AIDS-related cases escalated to epidemic proportions beneath the scenes of a fight for a democracy.
4. The passage of time: Precious time was lost since the initial HIV infections.
5. Denial of the reality of the HIV and AIDS epidemic.

---

[184] https://1ref.us/sp (accessed 5/6/2019).

"It was only post 1994 [that South Africa] 'suddenly began to face the fact that we had a huge number of people desperately ill and dying, including children.' And it was only much later that the country began to deal with the crisis." According to Bishop Dowling there was also an attitude of denial in the country. "So by the time we came together as a nation to deal with it, we had about 5 million people infected and dying."

3.5.1.2 Catholic Action and Responses to the HIV and AIDS Epidemic

- Active initiatives in the poor communities to lighten the burden of the scourge;
- Development of Home-Based Care projects;
- Funding of projects: The major change came when US President Bush's "Emergency Plan for AIDS Relief," called PEPFAR, in 2003 started to fund faith-based organizations involved in AidS programs providing antiretroviral drugs and supporting church-based programs.

3.5.1.3 Challenges the Catholic Church Faces

- The massive AIDS orphan problem.
- The increasing number of child-headed homes.
- The lack of ARVs.
- The increase in illegal settlements not serviced by the government—no schools or clinics.
- Lack of funding.

For decades the South African government and its people were more engaged in a fight against apartheid and in a struggling democracy, while hundreds were dying of AIDS-related illnesses daily.

3.5.1.4 *The Catholic Appeal in the Face of the HIV and AIDS Epidemic*[185]

- The appeal of the church goes out to Catholics for a stronger "commitment and relationship with Jesus, the inspiration we derive from the Gospel and the principles of Catholic Social Teaching which need to guide the actual creative practical responses we make on the ground."
- To "be pre-eminently engaged at the present time and going into the future—the holistic appreciation of the total social-cultural context of the AIDS orphans and child-headed households. Because that particular suffering, especially when it is linked to situations of extreme poverty, dehumanizes children in a terrible way, and takes away completely any hope they have of growing to the fullness that Jesus wants for them."
- To "be pre-eminently in programmes which try creatively and constructively to address that issue in the communities and with the communities. Working in relationship with our people in the communities, so they can be inspired by us, by our vision, by our principles. And with them "to look at what can we do, even with limited resources."

3.6   Findings

In this chapter it has become crystal clear that the HIV and AIDS epidemic is one of the fiercest challenges facing the Christian church in the twenty-first century in South Africa. All churches, Faith Based Organizations, faith communities of all persuasions, pastoral care and counselling, including all other ministries to PLWHA and affected by the epidemic, share in the overwhelming task of caring for the victims and survivors of the scourge of HIV infection and AIDS. Theology and theodicy[186] alike are being challenged. The fragility of human life and the value of the soul is challenged. Human identity is challenged. HIV and AIDS kill and destroy human dignity. For decades already this epidemic has been

---

[185] https://1ref.us/sp (accessed 5/6/2019).
[186] Philosophy dealing with the question of evil in the light of a good God.

a social malady of South African society taking millions of lives, with a thousand more dying each day.

How will we win the battle against the invasive and destructive HIV and AIDS epidemic is an all-consuming question in the face of an HIV and AIDS epidemic. This research is informed by the premise that the involvement and support of the Seventh-day Adventist Church in matters of HIV and AIDS is an imperative, and after a study on existing ecclesiologies and models in ministries to PLWHA, opts for an eclectic approach best suited and tailor-made for the Seventh-day Adventist Church to effective multidimensional Home-Based Care. Given the established pillars of her faith and the wealth of available established resources, the congregations of the Seventh-day Adventist Church in South Africa can initiate contextual Home-Based Care programs and projects, offering effective and compassionate pastoral care to PLWHA in poor communities.

I have greatly benefited by the following observations useful in planning the formulation of a Home-Based Care program:

1. Helderberg Hospice is a comprehensive palliative health care program for persons living with terminal illness and their families. The hospice included PLWHA in their daily program. I have gained vast experience, knowledge, and skill, which put me in the advantageous position to assist the Seventh-day Adventist Church with training and the launch of their own Home-Based Care program.
2. Ikhwezi is a government day hospital and clinic, a health care organization offering HIV, AIDS, and TB-related treatment, care and support services, and primary health care services to the community. This facility runs a well-functioning HIV and AIDS ARV clinic. As much as Ikhewzi Clinic is a government facility and not a FBO, I believe that the pastoral counsellor has the unique privilege to provide loving care to every patient regardless of their religious persuasion, background, race, or culture—every patient has the right to receive dignified treatment and respect. Every patient expects, longs for, and ought to be treated with dignity and care. This privileged

work provides the Christian counsellor and/or caregiver with the opportunity to be salt and light in the clinic and to bring Christ into every consultation, *living* the Word and bringing the presence of God closer to every patient.
3. While JL Zwane is owned and managed by the Presbyterian Church, its services are offered not only to its own members but also to the PLWHA and the families in the community. The Seventh-day Adventist Church would do well to consider the launch of a similar facility, especially in its poor communities.
4. While the Afro-Christian ministry approach provides adequate information for an Africa spirituality approach, the patriarchal paradigm in which it operates would place women and girls in a vulnerable position. Personally, therefore, I would not opt for this model in Home-Based Care.
5. Lastly, the Catholic Church model gives us tremendous evidence and insights into a very successful approach to Home-Based Care and highlights the all-round realities and challenges, which include the issues of women and children that such a program might encounter.

I would like to recommend that the Seventh-day Adventist Church network with various ecclesiologies operating Home-Based Care programs and projects to learn of the pros and the cons of a ministry of care to PLWHA in poor communities. I would also strongly suggest the Seventh-day Adventist Church use an eclectic approach to extract from the above models the aspects and applied methods that would help in the design and formulation of a Home-Based Care model tailor-made to suit the needs of their local church and local communities.

As a member of the Seventh-day Adventist Church I believe that the Church is a vital organ in the community and has the potential and capacity to mobilize their members at a grassroots level in the formation of localized CHBC programs in poor communities. Indeed, the Seventh-day Adventist Church is an integral part of the South African society, and being a church equipped for more than a century now with pillars in healthcare, education, printing and publishing, and medical missionary work, they have the capacity to:

- Initiate a successful Home-Based Care program in every poor community to cater effectively to PLWHA in the church and the community.
- Motivate and enlist all its members to volunteer in active ministries of care to PLWHA in their community.
- Design specific Home-Based care projects best suited for the local needs of PLWHA and ensure that such programmes and projects involve all departments[187] in the local church for ministries.
- Illustrate that the established Home-Based Care programs and projects be steered by the Health Ministries Department of the Church, under the auspices of the Personal Ministries Department, who will ensure and monitor that all other departments for ministry support and get on board the activities and services to PLWHA.
- And lastly, let the pastor, who is the shepherd, leader, and teacher and therefore the overseer, ensure that all members are encouraged and recruited for services and a compassionate ministry. The pastor and the Health Ministries Department should ensure that all members engaging as caregivers in Home-Based Care ministries receive adequate training, preparation, and empowerment for such for ministry.

Thus far, this research has pointed out the potential inherent in the doctrinal and practical legacy of the Seventh-day Adventist Church to design and formulate Home-Based Care programs suited to reach the PLWHA in poor communities. In the next and final chapter of this book there will be an attempt to formulate a theory of pastoral care and counselling to PLWHA within the Seventh-day Adventist context. Scripture models that can support such a theory will be discussed and proposed. A pastoral strategy will be provided and the potential inherent in the pillars

---

[187] Appendix #2: Departments.

of Adventist faith and healing for ministry to the PLWHA and their families will be developed. A Seventh-day Adventist model of Home-Based Care programs in the South African context of HIV and AIDS will be proposed, with recommendations and/or suggestions for how the Seventh-day Adventist Church can mobilize her members to support CHBC projects.

CHAPTER FOUR

The Seventh-day Adventist Church Within the Context of the HIV and AIDS Epidemic: Towards a Home-Based Care Model and Community-Focused Ecclesiology

4.1   Pastoral Care and Healthcare Ministries to PLWHA

Providing effective healthcare services and pastoral care to PLWHA in the South African context have become a tremendous challenge. An ever-increasing rate of 1,000 new infections daily of the HI virus, accessibility to ARV treatment, the quality level of service available, and scarce resources (all pointed out in Chapter One) are only a few of the numerous challenges of the HIV and AIDS epidemic in South Africa, the epicenter of a worldwide epidemic. PLWHA and their families are facing suffering, hardship, loss of family members, and grief on a daily basis. Thousands visit clinics or hospitals daily. Home-Based caregivers of several FBOs and communities of faith visit the sick and dying PLWHA to bring some comfort and relief, often in dire and harrowing situations. I believe that any faith-based community has a calling in this context and a moral responsibility to PLWHA. Moreover, with the combination of its health message and unique pillars of its faith, the Seventh-day Adventist Church in South Africa is positioned to make a huge difference in ministry to PLWHA here at the epicenter of an HIV and AIDS epidemic.

Pastoral care to PLWHA as one of the modalities through which faith-based communities are present has encountered challenges on different levels. This research has shown that spiritual care and counselling, therapy, practical and spiritual intervention, as well as empowerment of the community are all evidently challenged. The pastors and chaplains need help in caring for the increasing number of PLWHA in their congregations and their local communities. Evidently also, the lack of resources and overburdened pastors compound the issue even further. However, there are still vast opportunities for pastoral care in the field of HIV and AIDS in an ever-advancing HIV and AIDS epidemic in South Africa. Pastoral caregivers are usually welcomed with open arms in the homes of terminally ill patients, clinics, and hospitals. The support programs for staff and caregivers enhance their sense of calling to HIV and AIDS ministries and indirectly impact the quality of their service to patients. One of the biggest challenges is to create sustainable models for pastoral care and to equip caregivers and all stakeholders with adequate tools and skill to deal effectively with the challenges and opportunities they face in an HIV and AIDS ministry.

> "*Pastoral caregivers are usually welcomed with open arms in the homes of terminally ill patients, clinics, and hospitals.*"

This chapter is therefore an attempt to:

1. Provide a theological background that can be used to formulate a theory for pastoral caregiving within the context of the Seventh-day Adventist Church.
2. Formulate a theory for pastoral care and counselling to PLWHA and their families within the context of the Seventh-day Adventist Church.
3. Propose a model that can help Seventh-day Adventists to structure their Home-Based Care programs to PLWHA in answer to the research question: "How can the Seventh-day Adventist church model its Home-Based Care programs in the South African context and how

can it mobilize its members to support these Home-Based Care projects and initiatives?"
4. Provide a pastoral strategy for the implementation of the above praxis theory where the relevant pillars of the Adventist faith become the vehicles to reach the PLWHA and their families through healing ministries, intervention, education, and care.
5. Finally, recommend and suggest a way forward for Seventh-day Adventists in South Africa.

4.2 Pastoral Ministry and Care in a Multicultural Context: South Africa

We live and serve in a multicultural South African society. There is a great diversity of race, culture, and religions in South Africa. Unfortunately, traditions, culture, and religion can become barriers and hindrances to pastoral ministry and care. These barriers and hindrances must be faced and overcome, for South Africa is a country in crisis as far as the HIV and AIDS epidemic is concerned. If we don't manage the HIV and AIDS crisis in South Africa, then the crisis will manage us!

"If we don't manage the HIV and AIDS crisis in South Africa, then the crisis will manage us!"

People on the continent of Africa and the rest of the global community are desperately looking for answers. They are looking for meaning to their lives, meaning to their pain, and meaning to their suffering. Skilled pastoral counsellors can help individuals find the answers and help them to grow through their suffering, help them to successfully manage their disease, and in addition to that, look forward to a quality life and meaningful existence. The urgent need exists, therefore, for pastoral counsellors to enter into multicultural situations and effectively care for the people of Africa and South Africa. I am confident that the Seventh-day Adventist Church in South Africa has the potential but is in need of the help of established FBOs in setting up a ministry of contextual Home-Based Care to the PLWHA in South Africa.

When Jesus commissioned us to "go and make disciples of all nations,"[188] He also intended that His "house will be called a house of prayer [and healing] for all nations."[189] Paul, in His teaching on cross-cultural ministry, taught us that when in Rome he would be a Roman to the Romans, to the Jew he would be a Jew, and to the Gentile, a Gentile—that he might *"win those under the law"*[190] for God's kingdom. Therefore, to people in an African cultural context, pastoral care takes on an attitude of "I am an African."

This is by no means a dilution or a weakening of the gospel's power—the motive is to reach PLWHA wherever they are at their point of need, and care for them. To the pastoral counsellor and/or caregiver, this would mean befriending victims of disease, sickness, and suffering, and bringing healing to individuals for whom Christ died, thereby leading individuals to come and see and get to know the Great Physician.

The primary motivating factor for *doing* pastoral care is love—love for the person in need of care, that they might know and see who God, the *"I AM" Jehovah-Rophe*, is. What the world needs is Jesus—just a glimpse of Him who will bring joy for the sorrowful one and gladness, the healing balm in Gilead, to the suffering one. What PLWHA need is a true revelation of who God really is, and to be reconciled to Him, and to have renewed hope to live again. "Now this is eternal life: that they may know you, the only true God, and Jesus Christ, whom you have sent."[191] Lartey defines care as "the expression of spirituality in relation to self, others, God and creation."[192] Pastoral care is concerned with the exchange of care across barriers which have previously hindered expressions of empathy, love and justice. Pastoral care is the bridge across ethnic, religious and cultural boundaries to bring life, healing and hope to PLWHA from all walks of life. In Christ we are one. The prayer of Christ was and is that the

---

[188] Matthew 28:19, NIV.
[189] Mark 11:17, NIV.
[190] 1 Corinthians 9:20, NIV.
[191] John 17:3, NIV.
[192] Lartey (2003), 11.

Father would make all people one. In South Africa, a contextual Home-Based Care program will only be successful when a oneness of its people becomes a reality through aggressive intentional efforts of intercultural, cross-cultural or transcultural pastoral care—where Agape love in the heart of the pastoral caregiver in a ministry to PLWHA is indeed a revelation and answer to the prayer "Father make us one."

Lartey aptly cites Clebsch, Jaekle, and Pattison (1993) on their definition of pastoral care as pictured in "overtly theological language":

> Pastoral care is that activity, undertaken especially by representative Christian persons, directed towards the elimination and relief of sin and sorrow and the presentation of all people perfect in Christ to God.[193]

In my undergraduate degree I completed studies in intercultural communication and had to learn the skill of how to be sensitive and aware of the dynamics that are involved in the African contexts of culture, tradition, lifestyle practices, and worship styles—intercultural competence has to be learned, shared, taught, and lived. It is not something that happens automatically or comes naturally to the people of South Africa, especially those who are products of a segregated apartheid past. The wounds and scars of racial segregation run deep—trust among the races and the "skill" to live and work together are needed and the awareness of people's values, beliefs, and their understanding of God and who He is, is vital. It is important that we respect the views and the beliefs of all PLWHA. I believe that God can use the Seventh-day Adventist Church to bridge the existing gaps of racial divides, prejudice, stigmatization, and indifference—love for one's neighbor sees no race or skin color and therefore removes all stigma and prejudices through pastoral care.

I am an African by birth; more specifically, I am a South African citizen, but I have had to learn about the differentness and the many

---

[193] Lartey (2003), 23.

differences that made us, the people of South Africa, one great nation. Many unique differences exist among us when compared with the Western tradition. Totally different cultures, beliefs, rituals, norms, values, and lifestyle practices are involved and co-exist in the South African context. In the indigenous African mind-set, there is a totally distinct approach to disease, and managing physical challenges are more on a spiritual level than on the logical cause and effect level. A strong belief in the presence of the ancestors prevails—especially in times of illness, suffering, loss, distress, and death.

In true African tradition the concepts of disease, affliction, death, and dying have strong implications to the community, family, and the individual experiencing the crisis. It is vital that pastoral caregivers are cognizant of this.

> Africa is not as previously erroneously viewed as a pure world of harmony within wonderful relationships. Often the ubuntu principle is described as if Africa is still a rural country with peaceful relationships and that the only reason why we got problems is due to colonialism, slavery and racism. This is not the case. Such an approach is naïve and unrealistic.[194]

According to Prof. Daniël Louw, Africa is a philosophical concept, which describes a complexity and diversity of its people—the different cultural, local, and contextual settings related to a state of being and mind-set. The reference to Africa is an attempt to describe the unique contribution of the rich diversity of modes of being in Africa to a global world.

For me personally as a pastor, counsellor, and caregiver, the principles employed in pastoral counselling in a multicultural ministry to PLWHA are simple:

With Jesus Christ as the Great Example and Best Role Model:

---

[194] Louw, D. J. *Pastoral Care in an African Context.*

1. To study and to follow the methods Jesus employed;
2. To meet people where they are in their point of need and in their personal space and environment;
3. To befriend people (getting accustomed to their beliefs, norms and values—then respecting their value system as well as our own);
4. To meet their desperate and immediate needs and to care for them;
5. To build a relationship of trust and thereby warm their hearts and win their confidence (trust). Quality relationships in respect of religious powers, community prescriptions, and family customs are of vital importance;
6. Then, if they show an interest and are willing, to invite them to "Follow Him."

To people from differing belief systems it is important that the "foreigner" (any person from outside of the given culture) understands and respects them as people, as well as their value system that gave them a sense of being, of belonging, and taught them a good way of living.

I have gained extensive knowledge over time, and ministry in the African context has provided me with many insights into the African spirituality, worldview, and mind-set. The experience still yields new insights, and continuing ministry remains a privilege. There is always something new to learn in the African culture. One can never know it all or have it all. An open-minded approach to learning all there is to learn, and a willingness to "adopt" another's culture in order to be an effective minister of God's love and grace: this is the goal in pastoral care and counselling in an African context.

4.3 Important Considerations in an African Spirituality

- In the African context strong beliefs of spiritual powers and forces exist.
- Systems thinking and practice of patience. The total person must be cared for in a systematic environment. Traditionally the Africans hold to a group culture and therefore the total person belongs to a

group. The person is important as one part of a whole group/culture/community.
- An ever-present mystic dimension of life prevails, so in order for pastoral caregivers to reach the individual it is important to understand the patient's beliefs.
- Human agents cause sickness.
- The community is all important, before—and much more than—the individual.
- Evil, which has an influence on people's lives, is not merely an external factor. The cause of evil lies in the person.
- To be able to identify and understand the reasons for suspicion which underlie any aggressive behaviour.
- Group and community counselling become an essential part of therapy.
- The challenge is to cultivate a sense of solidarity, belonging, mutual love, affection, and unconditional acceptance.
- Spirituality in healing: meaning and destination is to be stressed.
- Aspects of restoration, retribution, and reconciliation—offering, sacrifice, and compensation—play an important role in regaining balance: Christ's sacrificial death as a bestowal of God's grace.
- Healing and life: The Biblical notion of *"Life"* energy and power as reconciliation must be communicated. The power of the resurrection normalizes life and offers a link to life after death.
- The church as family and system of relationships: The church is to be introduced as a *"body"* with *koinonia* ties.
- Rituals and symbols: The cross is a symbol of restored relationships.
- Serving Holy Communion is very important—it communicates support, grace, concern, love, reconciliation, and a sense of belonging. It helps the victim or the perpetrator to experience forgiveness.
- The pastor as listener and interpreter of stories—in a sense "prophet healer."
- Pedagogical and indirective counselling—the role of elders is very important.

– Interculturality within counselling: The skills of interpathy—the pastoral counsellor is an intercultural person, entering into a second culture.

It is imperative for a successful ministry of pastoral care in multicultural and pluralistic settings, that the pastor is sensitive and knowledgeable on how to *feed and tend* God's different and differing lambs from a caring, accommodating, loving, and compassionate heart. Therefore, from the theological perspective and Christian understanding, the pastoral caregiver needs to undergo a process of *kenosis*[195]—setting self aside or an emptying of oneself and experience the "adoption" of another's culture and worldview through "engaging acts of self-giving and care."

In every culture, regardless of how religion or spirituality is experienced and has shaped us, the pastoral expression of healing is rooted within these multidimensional relationships and, as such, illuminates the fundamental nature of life as radically relational.

In this world, sickness and diseases of all kinds including HIV and AIDS, suffering, grief, loss, pain, and death, are all part and parcel of the human experience, of the reality of daily life and existence. The HIV and AIDS epidemic has become a serious malady of the South African society, destroying millions of lives and wiping out the ideal family structure as God designed it to be for His glory.

4.4 The Scripture and Theological Background for Theory Formation

4.4.1 The Scripture and Pastoral Care as Home-Based Care

From the early part of the 19th century, the pioneer of the Adventist movement, Ellen G. White, saw the need for the Seventh-day Adventist Church to embrace the holistic approach to healing as a means of achieving its mission in the world.[196] Since then the Church traditionally has always

---
[195] Lartey, *In Living Color* (2003):175, 176.
[196] Okemwa (2003), 23.

looked at illness not only as physical distress but also as a spiritual distress, which needs to be addressed. From the scriptural point of view, the Seventh-day Adventist Church focuses on Jesus who is depicted as one who cured many diseases, helping those who were vulnerable. Indeed, the healing of the lepers and the outcasts brought about the restoration of their spiritual as well as their physical well-being, thus reinstating their human dignity and their status in the society. This shows that the Seventh-day Adventist Church in South Africa should be a place where agape love is expressed openly among Church members and PLWHA.

4.4.1.1 *Agape Love at the Heart of Pastoral Care*

Emmanuel Lartey is of the view that the heart of the "hiddenness" of pastoral care is love.[197] I am of the opinion that as a community of faith, the Seventh-day Adventist Church should demonstrate that Christ's love is the compelling force that drives a compassionate ministry of pastoral care to people living with HIV and AIDS. The love of Christ constrains us, compels us, and moves us! We love others and serve others through healing ministries because He first loved us.[198]

Jesus taught the important lesson of love for one's neighbor: "*If you love Me, keep My commandments.*"[199] He also reminded us that, "*Thou shalt love the Lord thy God with all thy heart, and with all thy soul, and with all thy mind ... thou shalt love thy neighbour as thyself.*"[200] This kind of true "love for God" should be seen in "love for neighbor" in a ministry of compassion, comfort, and care to PLWHA, as a reflection to the world of Christ in the heart, the hope of all glory to PLWHA. True fulfilling of, and true obedience to, the commands of God means to care for one's neighbor and to carry one another's burdens.

---

[197] Lartey (2003), 29.
[198] 1 John 4:19.
[199] John 14:15, NKJV.
[200] Matthew 22:36–39, KJV.

In the story of the Good Samaritan, a Pharisee, an expert of the Law, asked Jesus the greatest question ever asked: "Teacher … what must I *do* to inherit eternal life?"[201] Jesus gave this lawyer an opportunity to answer his own question and he answered rightly quoting the Scriptures on love for God and love for one's neighbor. But in an attempt to justify himself and hoping to escape the requirements of the Law, this expert of the Mosaic Law asked, "And who is my neighbor?"[202] The Pharisee clearly *knew* the whole Law. The rich young ruler in Mark 10:17–27 asked Jesus the same question, "What must I do to inherit eternal life?"[203] and asserted to have kept the law since childhood![204] The rich young ruler, however, was deceived as to his true condition. The heart of the Law is the agape love of its Author. In answer to the lawyer's question, "Who is my neighbor?" Jesus tells a story in Luke chapter ten that reveals the true nature of law-keeping. This story of the unfortunate man who travelled down from Jerusalem to Jericho is the relevant passage of Scripture for the Church today, and for pastoral care. The all-important question in this book is: "Where does the Seventh-day Adventist Church in South Africa position herself in the parable of the Good Samaritan?"

> "The love of Christ constrains us, compels us, and moves us! We love others and serve others through healing ministries because He first loved us."

4.4.1.2 The Good Samaritan: Pastoral Care as Love for Neighbor

In the parable of the Good Samaritan,[205] Jesus revealed the needs of one who suffers at the hand of a robber … beaten up, bruised, and left for dead on the Jericho road of life. He is injured, ill, hurt and in need of help

---

[201] Luke 10:25, NIV.
[202] Luke 10:29, NIV.
[203] Mark 10:17, NIV.
[204] Mark 10:20.
[205] Luke 10:25–37.

and healing—an unfortunate traveler on the Jericho road. In this parable Jesus also foretold the possible reactions and responses of the pastors, the priests, and the Levites among us as He pointed out the compassion shown by the Good Samaritan, whom the Jews hated, discriminated against, and looked upon with scorn and disdain. Commentators would have it that the injured man on the Jericho road was probably a Jew. What a serious indictment on the priest and the Levite in 21st century Adventism in the face of an HIV and AIDS epidemic. What a wakeup call to show love for our neighbors in need of pastoral care and a ministry of compassion.

The Seventh-day Adventist pastor is called upon to heed the Word of the Lord and to pay close attention the words of Jesus Christ in this parable, and in like fashion of the Good Samaritan, to dispel and discharge all possible existing prejudice and discrimination of PLWHA among their members, remove all such possible prejudices of stigmatization, and eradicate all possible marginalization and rejection of ones who fell into the hands of the robber. The work of the pastor is to care for the sick and the dying, to bring hope and healing to anxious sufferers. Pastoral care as Home-Based Care is a sacred charge of their duty to the sick and suffering, the lonely shut-ins, and victims of HIV and AIDS. It is the role and responsibility of the pastor to engage in the training of their members, and to equip the Church to be mobilized in structured ministries through Home-Based Care to PLWHA. Ultimately it is the role and calling of pastoral care to bring hope and healing—resurrection hope—to the sick and dying. Care of soul translates to cure of soul when effective pastoral care and counselling through Home-Based Care in the Seventh-day Adventist Church becomes a reality.

> The sound counsel to the Seventh-day Adventist Church is this: the work of gathering in the needy, the oppressed, the suffering, and the destitute, is the very work which every church that believes the truth for this time should long since have been doing. We are to show the tender sympathy of the Samaritan in supplying physical necessities,

feeding the hungry, bringing the poor that are cast out to our homes, gathering from God every day grace and strength that will enable us to reach to the very depths of human misery and help those who cannot possibly help themselves. In doing this work we have a favorable opportunity to set forth Christ the crucified One.[206]

4.4.1.3 Salt and Light Metaphors: Pastoral Care as Salt and Light

In Matthew chapter five, we find the "salt of the earth" and "light of the world" metaphors that occur as part of a discourse in Jesus' sermon on the mount. These very famous metaphors frequently used in Christian circles are crucial to this research in addressing the need for contextual Home-Based Care to PLWHA.

> *13 "You are the salt of the earth. But if the salt loses its saltiness, how can it be made salty again? It is no longer good for anything, except to be thrown out and trampled underfoot.*
>
> *14 "You are the light of the world. A town built on a hill cannot be hidden.*
>
> *15 Neither do people light a lamp and put it under a bowl. Instead they put it on its stand, and it gives light to everyone in the house.*
>
> *16 In the same way, let your light shine before others, that they may see your good deeds and glorify your Father in heaven."*[207]

Pastoral care cannot be successful and effective while functioning separate or aloof in the communities where the church exists. Both salt

---
[206] White, *Testimonies for the Church, Vol. 6*, 276.1.
[207] Matthew 5:13–16, NIV.

and light are commodities that play an essential role in daily human existence—both are necessary and we cannot do without them.

The church of God on earth, also known as the people of God or the followers of Jesus, are equated to salt and light: "You are the salt," and "You are the light." In this discourse Jesus is not asking whether His disciples are the salt, nor is He requesting of them to become the salt and the light. A careful study of the Scriptures shows us a state of "being":

The original Greek text is:

> Ὑμεῖς ἐστε τὸ ἅλας τῆς γῆς· ἐὰν δὲ τὸ ἅλας μωρανθῇ,
> ἐν τίνι ἁλισθήσεται; εἰς οὐδὲν ἰσχύει ἔτι
> εἰ μὴ βληθὲν ἔξω καταπατεῖσθαι ὑπὸ τῶν ἀνθρώπων.

The translation of the King James Bible reads:

> *Ye are the salt of the earth: but if the salt has lost his savour, wherewith shall it be salted? it is thenceforth good for nothing, but to be cast out, and to be trodden under foot of men.*

The World English Bible translates the passage as:

> *You are the salt of the earth, but if the salt has lost its flavor, with what will it be salted? It is then good for nothing, but to be cast out and trodden under the feet of men.*[208]

Salt and light are extremely important and the issue of salt losing its savour or flavour becomes problematic when it refers to the church of God on earth. By nature, salt (sodium chloride) is extremely stable and cannot lose its flavour. On the same score in the light metaphor, the followers of Christ are the ones who give light to the world and are likened to a city on a hill. Light dispels darkness and helps people find their way.

---

[208] https://1ref.us/sq (accessed 5/6/2019).

It is noteworthy that in John 9:5[209] Jesus Himself claims to be the light of the world and then in Matthew 5:14 He calls His disciples' attention to "You are the light." The application of the salt and light metaphors are crucial to authentic Christian living and twenty-first century ministry and Home-Based Care to PLWHA.

The above metaphors of salt and light speak of a moral philosophy and the moral fiber of society that will make a difference in the lives people. Jesus is our example and Jesus' method alone will make the salt and light model of the New Testament a saving reality of hope when the church of God on earth will "mingle with [people] as one who sought their good, befriended them and cared for their needs…"[210] When the people of God will mingle as "salt of the earth," then the "Light of the world" will become the light to all who are suffering and in darkness. Darkness fails to exist in the presence of light. Light dispels darkness and brings hope and healing to the sick, suffering soul.

The church of God ought not to hide their light under the bushel, but to let their light so shine before all people that their Father in Heaven will be lifted up and glorified, and draw men and women to Himself, saving all people from suffering, death, and destruction.

4.4.1.4 *Pastoral Care as "Immanuel, God with Us"*

Bringing the presence of God in the sick room means to create a space of grace for the patient. Creating an atmosphere of grace in the sick room is bringing the presence of God to the sick person and the possibility of hope for their healing. Often Jesus went into the homes of the sick person to minister to them. From the many biblical examples throughout Jesus' ministry on earth we find evidences of the Word taking on human form, becoming "flesh and dwelling among us."[211] They are the clear indications

---

[209] https://1ref.us/sr (accessed 5/6/2019).
[210] White, *Ministry of Healing*, 143.
[211] John 1:14, NIV.

of fulfillment of the Old Testament prophetic foretelling of *"Immanuel,"*[212] God with us—Christ, coming to seek and to save the lost and to meet with people at their point of need.

"For God sent *not his* Son into the world *to condemn the world*; but that the world through him might be saved."[213] After the Savior's ignominious death on the cross and His victorious resurrection, having been given all authority in heaven and earth, He gave the great commission to His eleven disheartened disciples, to "go and make disciples of all nations…" and to "teach them to obey everything [He] commanded [them]."[214] At the same time, He gave them the assurance "I am with you always, to the very end of the age."[215] This great commission is ours today, to go into the whole world, more specifically to the people of South Africa, and to bring the good news of the Gospel, healing, and deliverance from sin in the name of Jesus. This is the work of the church and the call to pastoral care. The great commission of our Lord was intended as an extension and a reflection of *"Immanuel, God with Us"* through ministries of grace.

4.5 Background for Theory Formation Continued: The Spirit of Prophecy—Ellen G. White and a Ministry of Compassion

First and foremost, before determining the relevance of the writings of Ellen G. White in a ministry of compassion, it is necessary to state that the worldwide Seventh-day Adventist Church holds as a doctrine *The Gift of Prophecy*[216] as:

> One of the gifts of the Holy Spirit is prophecy. This gift is an identifying mark of the remnant church and was

---

[212] Isaiah 7:14, NIV; Matthew 1:23, NIV.
[213] John 3:17, KJV, emphasis added.
[214] Matthew 28:19, NIV.
[215] Matthew 28:20, NIV.
[216] https://1ref.us/ss (accessed 5/6/2019).

manifested in the ministry of Ellen. G. White. As the Lord's messenger, her writings are a continuing and authoritative source of truth which provide for the church comfort, guidance, instruction, and correction. They also make clear that the Bible is the standard by which all teaching and experience must be tested.[217]

The Seventh-day Adventist Church believes that Ellen G. White (1827–1915) was an inspired author. Among her century-old written works of guidance, counsel, admonition, instruction, and warning messages are also her profound *Ministry of Healing* and *Counsels on Health*, *Acts of the Apostles*, and 130 more books and manuscripts, which the Seventh-day Adventist Church and ministers of other denominations have found invaluable in God's work.[218] I have consulted numerous books in searching for guidance on pastoral care and counselling and care of the sick in a ministry of compassion through contextual Home-Based Care in South Africa and am confident that, having followed the counsels of Ellen G. White, many a victim of illness and disease can find comfort, healing and salvation in Christ.

> Every church member should feel it their special duty to labor for those living in their neighborhood. Study how you can best help those who take no interest in religious things. As you visit your friends and neighbors, show an interest in their spiritual as well as in their temporal welfare. Present Christ as a sin-pardoning Saviour. Invite your neighbors to your home, and read with them from the precious Bible and from books that explain its truths. This, united with simple songs and fervent prayers will touch their hearts. Let church members educate themselves to do this work. This is just as

---

[217] Fundamental Belief 18.
[218] Joel 2:28, 29; Acts 2:14–21; Heb. 1:1–3; Rev. 12:17; 19:10.

essential as to save the benighted[219] souls in foreign countries. While some feel the burden of souls afar off, let the many that are at home feel the burden of precious souls around them and work just as diligently for their salvation.[220]

1. Sound counsel is given that,

   > The hours so often spent in amusement that refreshes neither body nor soul should be spent in visiting the poor, the sick, and the suffering, or in seeking to help someone who is in need. … Men and women of God, persons of discernment and wisdom, should be appointed to look after the poor and needy, the household of faith first. These should report to the church and counsel as to what should be done.[221]

2. Education and economic empowerment of PLWHA, their families, and even teenaged children acting in child-headed homes are vital to a multi-faceted ministry:

   > Instead of encouraging the poor to think that they can have their eating and drinking provided free or nearly so, we should place them where they can help themselves. We should endeavour to provide them with work, and if necessary teach them how to work. Let the members of poor households be taught how to cook, how to make and mend their own clothing, how to care properly for the home. Let boys and girls be thoroughly taught some useful trade or occupation. We are to educate the poor to become self-reliant. This will be true help, for it will not only make them self-sustaining, but will enable them to help others.[222]

---

[219] *Benighted*: in a state of pitiful or contemptible intellectual or moral ignorance.
[220] White, *Testimonies for the Church, Vol. 6*, 276.2.
[221] White, *Testimonies for the Church, Vol. 6*, 276.3, 278.4.
[222] White, *Testimonies for the Church, Vol. 6*, 278.5.

3. Pastoral care is deliberate action to reach people in all walks of life and to engage every church member. The efforts of all are needed. It is important that the purposes of God are presented to the members:

> It is God's purpose that the rich and the poor shall be closely bound together by the ties of sympathy and helpfulness. He bids us interest ourselves in every case of suffering and need that shall come to our knowledge.[223]

4. The privilege of the dignified work to PLWHA is a sacred duty of pastoral care. Ellen G. White counsels:

> Think it not lowering to your dignity to minister to suffering humanity. Look not with indifference and contempt upon those who have laid the temple of the soul in ruins. These are objects of divine compassion. He, who created all, cares for all. Even those who have fallen the lowest are not beyond the reach of His love and pity. If we are truly His disciples, we shall manifest the same spirit. The love that is inspired by our love for Jesus will see in every soul, rich or poor, a value that cannot be measured by human estimate. Let your life reveal a love that is higher than you can possibly express in words.[224]

5. I have had the experience in clinical work that not many patients may respond positively at first to Christian counsellors. However, the importance of persevering in a labor of love cannot be overemphasized:

> I have been instructed that the medical missionary work will discover, in the very depths of degradation, individuals who, though they have given themselves up to intemperate living and harmful habits, will respond to the right kind of labor. But they need to be recognized and encouraged.

---

[223] White, *Testimonies for the Church, Vol. 6*, 279.1.
[224] White, *Testimonies for the Church, Vol. 6*, 279.2.

Firm, patient, earnest effort will be required in order to lift them up. They cannot restore themselves. They may hear Christ's call, but their ears are too dull to take in its meaning; their eyes are too blind to see anything good in store for them. They are dead in trespasses and sins. Yet even these are not to be excluded from the gospel feast. They are to receive the invitation: "Come." Though they may feel unworthy, the Lord says: "Compel them to come in." Listen to no excuse. By love and kindness lay right hold of them. "Ye, beloved, building up yourselves on your most holy faith, praying in the Holy Ghost, keep yourselves in the love of God, looking for the mercy of our Lord Jesus Christ unto eternal life. And of some have compassion, making a difference: and others save with fear, pulling them out of the fire." (Jude 20–23)[225]

6. Often individuals might not respond positively to caregivers and hearts will harden under loving rebuke, "but they cannot withstand the love expressed toward them in Christ." We should encourage the sinner "not to feel himself an outcast from God" and encourage them to "look to Christ, who alone can heal the soul leprous with" the results of sin. "Reveal to the desperate, discouraged sufferer that he is a prisoner of hope. Let your message be: 'Behold the Lamb of God, which taketh away the sin of the world.'"[226]

7. "This work" of a ministry of compassion if:

> properly conducted, will save many a poor sinner who has been neglected by their churches. Many not of our faith are longing for the very help that Christians are in duty bound to give. If God's people would show a genuine interest in their neighbors, many would be reached by the

---

[225] White, *Testimonies for the Church, Vol. 6*, 279.4.
[226] White, *Testimonies for the Church, Vol. 6*, 279.3.

special truths for this time. Nothing will or ever can give character to the work like helping the people just where they are. Thousands might today be rejoicing in the message if those who claim to love God and keep His commandments would work as Christ worked."[227]

8. "When the medical missionary work thus wins men and women to a saving knowledge of Christ and His truth, money and earnest labor may safely be invested in it, for it is a work that will endure."[228]

When taking a closer look at Christ's method, it's like looking into a mirror, doing an evaluation and seeing the "flaws" of the church. As pastors, we can immediately detect our problem in ministry. Too often and for too long the focus of ministry has been only on making disciples and baptizing people, while scores are suffering and dying a Christ-less death. A ministry and service of disinterested benevolence is needed and Jesus is our Greatest Example. The Saviour mingled and interacted with people. He met them where they were, at their point of need. The motivation was to take care of their needs and to minister to them by taking care of their physical needs, often feeding and daily healing them. He desired their good and had their best interest at heart. He showed sympathy for their suffering and attended to their needs. While caring for human needs, the Saviour won their trust and confidence. He got to know them and they knew He was sincere in caring for them. The record shows us repeatedly in the Word of God that Christ's invitation to follow Him, came after He won their trust.

Stigmatization, discrimination, condemnation, marginalization, judgmentalism, and rejection were not on Jesus' daily agenda. Christ had no selfish ambition or ulterior motivation—He mingled with people as to reveal the love of the Father. **Charity** (agápē, Greek: ἀγάπη), which is altruistic in nature, is the *love* that serves regardless of changing humanity's

---

[227] White, *Testimonies for the Church, Vol. 6*, 280.1.
[228] White, *Testimonies for the Church, Vol. 6*, 280.2.

reactions and responses to His love. The message of the Gospel is a message of hope and of God's agape love to the people.[229]

Jesus Christ's method alone will give us success in a ministry of the highest form of love, and of hope and healing to the people of South Africa living with HIV and AIDS and all affected. When these strategic principles of Christ are employed, our success in pastoral care and the resulting blessings and rewards are guaranteed. Through Christ's method the love of God will be revealed in the Lord and a reverence for God will return to the world.

In her book *The Ministry of Healing*, Ellen G. White wrote the following:

> When Christ sent forth the disciples with the gospel message, faith in God and His word had well-nigh departed from the world. Among the Jewish people, who professed to have a knowledge of Jehovah, His word had been set aside for tradition and human speculation. Selfish ambition, love of ostentation, greed of gain, absorbed men's thoughts. As reverence for God departed, so also departed compassion toward men. Selfishness was the ruling principle, and Satan worked his will in the misery and degradation of mankind.[230]

Pastoral care is sharing God's love with the PLWHA and having a return of God's love and reverence for God in the world in instances where love is lacking or has failed and grown cold. Ultimately, this is true obedience to the gospel's call and living in obedience to the commandments of God means: "If you love Me, Keep My commandments."[231] The commandments of God could be summed up as two:

---

[229] **Agape** (/ˈæɡəpiː/ or /ˈæɡəpɪ/; Classical Greek: ἀγάπη, agápē; Modern Greek: αγάπη IPA: [aˈɣapi]), translated as "**love**: the highest form of **love**, especially brotherly **love**, charity; the **love** of God for man and of man for God." https://1ref.us/st (accessed 5/6/2019).

[230] White, *The Ministry of Healing*, 142.

[231] John 14:15, NKJV.

1. *Love for God, and*
2. *Love for neighbors.*

When pastoral care is understood as the sharing God's love with the PLWHA, it also means that pastoral care becomes the *comfort of God*—providing adequately for the healthy sheep of the flock who are safely in the fold, but more especially meeting the lost and injured lambs (PLWHA) of the flock where they were, even to the extent of going in search after/for them. Comfort of God brings the presence of God in the truest sense of the Word to the PLWHA.

4.6   Pastoral Care as "Comfort of God"—PAV Psalm 23[232]

Inasmuch as the salt and light, the Good Samaritan discussed above and *Immanuel*, "God with us" metaphors discussed in chapter two are beneficial instruments in pastoral care and counselling, the vital importance in a ministry of compassion to PLWHA cannot be overemphasized. PLWHA and their families stare death in the face daily and experience the turmoil of soul-destroying existential threats[233] acting as immunity viruses breaking down the life forces, e.g., anxiety, loss and rejection, guilt and shame, doubt and despair, helplessness and vulnerability, frustration, disillusionment, and anger. The parable of the Good Shepherd as comfort of God is the highest form of the expression of grace towards sinners and suffering humanity. When God as the loving and caring Good Shepherd is presented to PLWHA they experience the comfort of God as a healing balm for the soul in the assurance that He cannot crush the bruised reed.[234] On the same score the pastor will in like manner extend God's grace to the victim of HIV and AIDS in their care, introducing the vulnerable, sick, or

---

[232] Mathers, Arnet C. *The Shepherd's Psalm 23 (PAV)*. Calais, Maine (2015). https://1ref.us/su (accessed 5/6/2019).

[233] Daniël Louw's theory on existential threats as viruses of the soul will be extensively discussed in chapter four.

[234] Matthew 12:20.

dying person to the Good Shepherd as Jehovah Jireh, the great Provider for their every physical and spiritual need.

Psalm 23

1. Psalm of David
   YHWH[i] [is] my Shepherd,
      [Consequently[ii]]
         * I will not lack [anything].
2. * In pastures [full[iii]] of new-fresh-grass
      He will cause/allow me to lie down,
   * To waters tranquil
      He will carefully escort[iv] me.
3. * My soul He will revive.[v]
   * He will lead me in well-beaten paths[vi] of righteousness
      For the sake of His name/reputation.
4. * Even if[vii] I were walking in the valley of shadow of death,
      I would not fear evil.
        For
          You [are] with me,
            Your rod (of rulership[viii]) and Your staff (for support[ix]),
          They will comfort/encourage me.
5. * You will prepare before my face a table
      in front of my attackers [and they will be helpless to prevent it].
      You have anointed with oil my head.
      My cup [is] over-abundance.
6. * Surely,
      Goodness and steadfast-faithful-graciousness[x]
        will pursue me all the days of my life, and
      I will dwell in the house of YHWH to the end of days.[x][235]

---

[235] The footnotes for Psalm 23 (PAV):

i. "YHWH" is the holy name of God, referred to as the *tetragrammaton* (four letters). It is generally translated LORD because the oral tradition preserved in the Masoretic text is *'Adonai* or "lord." The word *Jehovah* comes from trying to fit the vowels of the oral tradition

Ellen G. White provides this powerful definition of grace:

> Grace is an attribute of God exercised toward undeserving human being. We did not seek for it, but it was sent in search of us. God rejoices to bestow His grace on us, not because we are worthy, but because we are so utterly unworthy. Our only claim to His mercy is our great need.[236]

---

written beneath the *tetragrammaton* by the Masoretes with the four Hebrew consonants YHWH of the written tradition.

ii. "...[T]he prefix conjugation [imperfect conjugation] may represent a future situation as dependent or contingent on some other expressed or unexpressed situation...." Waltke, B. K., & O'Connor, M. P. (1990). *An Introduction to Biblical Hebrew Syntax* (p. 512). Winona Lake, IN: Eisenbrauns.

iii. "*N'oth deše'* Ps 23:2 (full of grass, cf. Akk. *pargāniš* in the green meadow, AHw. 833a)" Koehler, L., Baumgartner, W., Richardson, M. E. J., & Stamm, J. J. (1999). *The Hebrew and Aramaic lexicon of the Old Testament* (electronic ed., p. 679). Leiden; New York: E.J. Brill.

iv. "to **escort**, with care, with *'al* to water Ps 23:2." *The Hebrew and Aramaic lexicon of the Old Testament* (electronic ed., p. 675).

v. "to refresh, restore the soul Ps 23:3, literally 'to bring back liveliness, vitality.' (Kraus *Ps.* 33:8)" *The Hebrew and Aramaic lexicon of the Old Testament* (electronic ed., p. 1431).

vi. **waggon track, firm path** Ps 65:12." *The Hebrew and Aramaic lexicon of the Old Testament* (electronic ed., p. 609).

vii. "The particle *ki* can also introduce an irreal conditional (Psalm 23:4)." Waltke, B. K., & O'Connor, M. P. (1990). *An introduction to biblical Hebrew syntax* (p. 638). Winona Lake, IN: Eisenbrauns.

viii. "**rod**: •a. α) in general; β) a rod with which to beat out cummin seed; γ) a rod as a weapon; δ) a rod as an instrument of punishment; •b) the shepherd's staff; •c) the rod, or cane, of an instructor (also used by God); •d) the rod, sceptre of the ruler; •e) staff, rod, cane of God's discipline; •f) rod, sceptre." *The Hebrew and Aramaic lexicon of the Old Testament* (electronic ed., pp. 1388–1389).

ix. "**support, staff**: • for the sick Ex 21:19, the aged Zech 8:4, rulers Nu 21:18, angel Ju 6:21; • → 2K 4:29, 31; 18:21; Is 36:6; Ezk 29:6; Ps 23:4 (parallel with *šebet*—rod). †" *The Hebrew and Aramaic lexicon of the Old Testament* (electronic ed., p. 651).

x. "1. **joint obligation** between relatives, friends, host and guest, master and servant; • closeness, solidarity, **loyalty**; 2. in God's relationship with the people or an individual, **faithfulness, goodness, graciousness**" *The Hebrew and Aramaic lexicon of the Old Testament* (electronic ed., p. 336–337).

xi. "2. (temporally) length of life, long life Dt 30:20; Ps 21:5; 23:6; 91:16; 93:5; Jb 12:12; Pr 3:2, 16; La 5:20" *The Hebrew and Aramaic lexicon of the Old Testament* (electronic ed., p. 88).

The PAV (Pastor Arnet Version) October 22, 2015.

[236] White, *The Ministry of Healing*, 161.2.

When the pastor as a person has experienced the *encounter of God's grace* in the personal sinful condition, then they are best able to extend this same grace to all whom the world may deem as undeserving of mercy. Ellen G. White counsels that God "through Jesus Christ holds out His hand all day long in invitation to the sinful and fallen. He will receive all. He welcomes all. It is His glory to pardon the chief of sinners. He will take the prey from the mighty, He will deliver the captive, He will pluck the brand from the burning fire. He will lower the golden chain of His mercy to the lowest depths of human wretchedness, and lift up the debased soul contaminated with sin."[237] Ultimately, this picture of God's grace as the loving, caring, and merciful Good Shepherd is the greatest model metaphor for effective pastoral care and counselling.

As shepherds of the flock of God—both inside and outside of the household of faith—the imperative is that the heart of the pastor…

> be linked with the hearts of those under his[her] charge. Let him[her] remember that they have many temptations to meet. We little realize the objectionable traits of character given to the youth as a birthright, and how often temptation comes to them as a result of this birthright.[238]

In an attempt to urge pastors and gospel workers in becoming good shepherds themselves under the leading and guidance of the Good Shepherd, also thereby giving us the exemplary pattern to behold, Ellen G. White further expounds on the vision shown her of the Good Shepherd:

> The guarding care that the under-shepherd will give the lambs of his[her] flock is well illustrated by a picture I have seen representing the Good Shepherd. The shepherd is leading the way, while the flock follow closely

---

[237] White, *The Ministry of Healing*, 161.
[238] White, *Gospel Workers*, 211.2.

behind. Carried in his arms is a helpless lamb, while the mother walks trustingly by his side. Of the work of Christ, Isaiah says, "He shall gather the lambs with His arm, and carry them in His bosom."[239] The lambs need more than daily food. They need protection, and must constantly be guarded with tender care. If one goes astray, it must be searched for. The figure is a beautiful one, and well represents the loving service that the under-shepherd of the flock of Christ is to give to those under his protection and care.

The metaphor of the Good Shepherd is the epitome of pastoral care and the highest form of leading the sick person into an encounter with God and the introduction to the *koinonia* fellowship of the household of faith and the kingdom of God. We are living in the time of earth's history with maladies of an end-time generation where the Seventh-day Adventist Church should redeem the time and possible wasted years when we should have been caring effectively for the sick in our churches and our communities. If we would follow Jesus, the Good Shepherd, as our greatest example, we would leave the ninety-nine good sheep and go in search of the anxious lost lambs of the household of faith and also the lost homeless lambs longing for the loving embrace of the Good Shepherd.

> Come near to them by personal effort. Evil invites them on every hand. Seek to interest them in that which will help them to live the higher life. Do not hold yourself aloof from them. Bring them to the fireside; invite them to join you around the family altar. Let us remember the claim of God upon us to make the path to heaven bright and attractive.[240]

---

[239] Isaiah 40:11.
[240] White, *Gospel Workers*, 212.

I value this contribution of the PAV translated version of Mathers giving fresh and new insights into the Good Shepherd's providences and loving, gracious, caring heart for the vulnerable lambs of the flock.

The assumption in this research study is, that in spite of the tremendous increase in knowledge and the great advances globally with phenomenal successes in the fields of medicine and technology, including the rapid discoveries in professional health-care services over the years, the challenges associated with human suffering and disease still seem insurmountable, especially in the context of the global HIV and AIDS epidemic.

4.7 Louw's Theological Reframing of Power: *Cura Vitae*: Power Tools in Pastoral Care as a Way Forward in Theory Formation in Contextual Home-Based Care to PLWHA in South Africa

I spent a whole year of structured course work in pastoral care and counselling, and have benefited tremendously from the teachings of Professor Daniël Louw, who is an icon in practical theology. More so, I have applied the theories and paradigms of Prof. Louw in pastoral care with amazingly positive results and am therefore completely certain that Prof. Louw's theories and models are helpful to Seventh-day Adventists and effective tools in Home-Based Care ministries among the people of South Africa. Seventh-day Adventists have had sound doctrine and good structures in place for decades already, but unless they follow practical methods to reach PLWHA, their pillars of faith will prove futile. "[W]hatever you did for one of the least of these brothers and sisters of Mine, you did for Me"—Jesus (Matthew 25:40, NIV).

Cura Vitae: Cure and care of soul as life care—Providing effective health care services and pastoral care to PLWHA in the South African context has become a tremendous challenge. Pastoral care to PLWHA as one of the modalities through which faith-based communities are present has encountered several challenges on different levels in South Africa. Prof. Daniël Louw has successfully designed *A Pastoral Hermeneutics of*

Care and Encounter: A Theological Design for a Basic Theory, Anthroplogy, Method and Therapy[241] and has developed a valuable theological model of *Cura Vitae in Illness and the Healing of Life*: soul cure and care as life care from the perspective of a Christian spirituality, with life dimensions of healing, which I have found extremely beneficial and effective in pastoral care, more especially in my ministry to PLWHA in the context of an African spirituality in South Africa. I would therefore recommend that the Seventh-day Adventist Church consider Prof. Louw's theological reframing of power: *Cura Vitae* as a possible tool towards a new ecclesial direction in pastoral care.

Every Seventh-day Adventist church in the communities where they serve should bring relief to the burden of poverty, helplessness, and shame, and empower vulnerable family members, especially children, of PLWHA. Through offering training in social skills and life skills, and more particularly Home-Based Care training programs for their members, they can empower families of PLWHA with "finding and using resources outside of [themselves], in such a way as to enable them to think and act in ways that will result in greater freedom and participation in the life of the societies of which they are a part."[242] As much as *empowering the poor* might have become a slogan around the world, in South Africa the increasing poverty as a result of the HIV and AIDS epidemic is a reality that cannot be ignored. The Seventh-day Adventist Church can therefore serve as agents of compassionate caring ministries that will bring healing to poor communities.

Prof. Louw's theory of *Cura Vitae*, as healing of life of communities affected by the HIV and AIDS epidemic is essential to the current policy of the Seventh-day Adventist Church. Theoretically, the church has a good policy on HIV and AIDS in place. However, the workload of district pastors where the ratio of pastors to churches is enormous,

---

[241] Louw, D. J. (1998).
[242] Lartey (2003), 68.

renders managing their PLWHA in the church and the communities an impossible task.

Traditionally, the pastors would visit the sick in their homes or in hospitals and medical facilities where they receive treatment. It is often the case in the poorer communities that pastors are assigned to many congregations in their care. The widespread pervasiveness of the HIV and AIDS epidemic in situations like these has become challenging for the local pastor as sole caregiver for the sick members in their congregations, as well as PLWHA in the communities. District pastors need the help of their church members, including volunteers, in local communities to aid in caring for the sick and the poor.

A paradigm shift is therefore needed from the traditional way of doing pastoral care for the sick to the notion of Home-Based Care to PLWHA. Pastors should equip and empower their members and ablebodied PLWHA to help carry the burden of care. *Cura Vitae* is a necessary and powerful tool to help pastors identify the existential threats as viruses of the soul that rob the poor, the sick, suffering person of life's vitality, and that impact on their relationship with God the Creator. When the body is sick, then the soul is sick; when the body suffers, the soul suffers. Often the presence of disease is as a result of a departure from the Creator's laws of healthful living. *Cura Vitae* is a comprehensive guide to assist the pastor with existential understanding and the appropriate development of skill to deal with illness, and lead the patient towards meaning in suffering, spiritual growth, and faith in God.

> The world is sick, and wherever the children of men[humans] dwell, suffering abounds. On every hand there is a seeking for relief. It is not the Creator's purpose that mankind shall be weighed down with a burden of pain, that his[their] activities shall be curtailed by illness, that his[their] strength wane, and his[their] life be cut short by disease … There is a need for an understanding of the

> many contributing factors to true happiness ... When sickness comes, it is essential that we employ the varied agencies which, in co-operation with nature's efforts, will build up the body and restore the health. There is, also, a larger more vitally important question—that of our relationship to the Creator who originally gave man[kind] [their] life, who made every provision for their continued happiness, and who today is interested in his[their] welfare.[243]

Throughout the Scriptures we find that there is a connection between poverty, illness, suffering, and sin. Jesus Christ came to our world to care for humanity's predicament and needs. In quoting the prophet Isaiah, Matthew clearly states: He "took up our infirmities and bore our diseases,"[244] in order to "minister to every need of humanity. The burden of disease and wretchedness and sin He came to remove."[245] Christ's compassion knew no limits. More than century ago Ellen G. White wrote the following: "The world needs today what it needed nineteen hundred years ago—a revelation of Christ. A great work of reform is demanded, and it is only through the grace of Christ that the work of restoration, physical, mental, and spiritual, can be accomplished."[246] This definitely is the great work of pastoral care which is desperately needed in the world *today*.

When the body suffers, then the soul is threatened with disease and death, and a deep longing and desire springs up in the heart of the sick person for God the Creator. The soul has been created to long for God its Maker—and "it is God's design that this longing of the human heart should lead to the One who alone is able to satisfy."[247] That longing is the soul sensing its need for healing and restoration. It is the privileged work and solemn responsibility that accompanies the call of pastors to

---

[243] White, *The Ministry of Healing*, 7.
[244] Matthew 8:17 (NIV).
[245] White, *The Ministry of Healing*, 17.1.
[246] White, *The Ministry of Healing*, 143.2.
[247] Publishers, preface to *The Desire of Ages* (Nampa, ID: Pacific Press Publishing Association, 1998).

communicate the good news of the gospel, the "good tidings to the poor; …to heal the broken-hearted…and to proclaim the year of the Lord's favour; [and thereby] …to comfort all those who mourn as God has commanded us in His Word."[248]

> When the gospel is received in its purity and power, it is a cure for the maladies that originated in sin. The Sun of Righteousness arises, "with healing in His wings."[249] Not all that the world bestows can heal a broken heart, or impart peace of mind, or remove care, or banish disease. Fame, genius, talent – all are powerless to gladden the sorrowful heart or to restore the wasted life. The life of God in the soul is man[kind's] only hope.[250]

Before further discussion of a need for *Cura Vitae* we will briefly look at coping with illness as an art.

4.8 Training Caregivers to Help PLWHA in Coping with Illness as an Art

Before any faith-based organization can embark in an effective Home-Based Care ministry essential training must take place. It is necessary that pastors prepare their members for dealing with the crisis of illness and death. It is important that pastors and caregivers view the patient's predicament of being ill as an opportunity for their spiritual growth. Prof. Louw asserts that:

> coping with illness becomes an art when patients succeed in viewing their illness as a very special opportunity for growth and that illness creates a new understanding of our

---
[248] Isaiah 61:1–3, Author paraphrase.
[249] Malachi 4:2.
[250] White, *The Ministry of Healing*, 115.2.

calling in life, a new understanding of our calling to represent the loving God of care in the world and become involved in the suffering of others.[251]

Earlier in this chapter the phenomenon of having been saved to serve and save others was highlighted in the salt, light, and Good Samaritan metaphors. The pastor is best positioned to empower patients and their families to practice the art of coping with illness as:

1. Putting meaning to suffering;
2. Trusting while everything seems futile; and
3. Living in the face of death.

Healing and survival "competency" therefore are borne out of the people's resilience and perceptive ability to transcend the existential threats such as fear and anxieties which accompany the challenge of being ill and to treat the crisis (pathology) as an opportunity for growth. According to Prof. Louw, the crisis of illness can be an opportunity for growth in life skills and faith, depending on the patient's framework of meaning, perception of life, and understanding of God (God-images).[252]

In order to help people to cope spiritually with illness, Prof. Louw's theory of God-images can help us understand the experience of the patient in a ministry of Home-Based Care to PLWHA. In Scripture we find several instances where, after Jesus delivered people from sin and healed the sick in communities, He encouraged them to show the same mercy and compassion, thereby sending them out to go and do the same. The disciples of Jesus Christ are the best example. Jesus Christ taught His disciples by His example in ministry. Not unless pastors have good knowledge and skill in pastoral care are they able to teach and impart knowledge to their members. Training is an essential and important

---

[251] Louw (2008), 10.
[252] Louw (2008), 9.

part of successfully equipping lay members. One of the major goals in pastoral ministry is to empower members to share in healing ministries. Another empowering tool in ministry to PLWHA is the concept of God-images. The concept of God-images helps the pastoral caregiver to assess the patient's view and understanding of God and is able to assess the patient's relationship with God and how they perceive God to be. This, therefore, is a useful approach to counselling the PLWHA in non-threatening ways.

4.9 God-images in Spiritual Healing

Spiritual maturity plays a vital role in dealing with poverty and managing illness and disease. The sufferer's relationship with God and their view of God determines their responses in their plight for survival and in the crisis of illness, suffering and death. *How people understand God and meaning in suffering becomes a pastoral problem.* Theodicy and God's involvement in suffering becomes an important factor to the sick person and their families. In Prof. Louw's theory of pastoral care he provides us a hermeneutics in care and counselling that helps pastors and caregivers with a diagnostic tool which is both useful in Home-Based Care and in the effective assessment of the patient's relationship and understanding of God.

> [S]piritual health within the pastoral model refers to the quality and nature of one's maturity in faith, which is determined by one's understanding of God. In a pastoral model images and conceptions of God play a decisive role in the 'healthy' functioning of mature faith. A pastoral assessment of health and sickness is not so much about correct or incorrect understanding, or good or bad concept. It is not about the doctrine of the church or the content of specific denominational confessions. It is about whether the concepts are appropriate or inappropriate

in terms of spiritual and life issues regarding our human quest for meaning and dignity.[253]

It is important to note that inappropriate God-images can lead to pathology and "spiritual illness" as well as to physical illness, disease, and discouragement. Therefore, fixed dogmatic ideas about morality and law connected with God and His will can lead to legalistic attitudes and undue austerity. An example where inappropriate perceptions of God can cause spiritual pathology is in situations where male violence relies on the underlying assumptions of patriarchy and the dominant role of control it affords males in the system, while images of a dominant male god prevail in the subconscious mind. In the South African society, most cultures adhere to patriarchy. Also, in the apartheid era, some churches presumed upon theological justifications for the ideology of racism. Pastoral caregivers must be aware that there is more than just one fixed view of God—that there are multiple paradigms simultaneously valid and useful. Pastoral care is not concerned with "correctness" or "incorrectness" of the patient's conception of God.

Prof. Louw states that, "Appropriate God-images denote existential and functional understandings and perceptions about God as related to the basic existential issues."[254]

Prof. Louw further proposes four main metaphoric models of God as concepts of God correlate with metaphors in Scripture and with specific contexts and situations.

---

[253] Louw (2008), 92.
[254] Louw (2008), 93.

God-image	Symbol	Effect
Monarchical Model: Sovereign, Ruler, King, Manager, Patriarch, Judge of history	Punishment, distance, apathy, power	Guilt or guilty feelings, self-discovery, self-examination, empowerment
Family Model: Father, Mother	Protective, pedagogic, caring, compassionate, guide, helper, provider, caregiver	Purification, growth, faith, education, meaning, *koinonia*
Covenantal Model: Savior, Redeemer, Friend	Compassion, confidant, companion, ally, mediation	Comfort, security, hope
Personal Model: Bridegroom, Helper, Advocate, Savior	Love, forgiveness, relationship	Acceptance, reconciliation, reinstatement, salvation

Figure 2: God-images: Symbols with Corresponding Concepts of God and Possible Effects

4.9.1 Four Metaphors: God-images

1. *The Monarchical Model*: God functions strongly as sovereign, ruler, king, manager, patriarch, judge of history—"omnipotence" features strongly, primarily as a dominant, militaristic, pantokrator, and/or force.

    The pastoral healer will communicate and translate the omnipotence of a God who reveals Himself as a vulnerable power of grace and compassion involved in the covenantal history of salvation. Omnipotence is then understood as a description of the manner in which God operates: His compassion, mercy, tenderness, His faithfulness and steadfastness, majesty, and His covenantal love.

2. *The Family Model*: God functions strongly as Father who is protective, and/or is pedagogic or as Mother who is caring and compassionate. God as Parent is actively involved with, and cares for his/her children. This God-image unites believers into one large family: *koinonia*, community of believers. Here the dominant image: God is guide, helper, provider, and caregiver.

3. *The Covenantal Model*: God is esteemed as the living God who intervenes in human history. A God who acts and intervenes in the interest of His children. God as confidant and companion, an ally and a Friend is the dominant image.
4. *The Personal Model*: God is seen within a network of a loving relationship in which different metaphors appear, e.g. the bridegroom, helper, advocate, and Saviour. The dominant image here is God as Beloved (God is Love, the Source and Origin of Love), and God as Saviour is a God who forgives and saves.

In the assessment of the patient, these metaphoric God-images and *Cura Vitae* models put "handles" on a pastoral diagnosis of spiritual maturity, and are therefore helpful in making pastoral relevant and successful in a Home-Based Care ministry.

In the application of a pastoral model for the development of a mature faith an interaction of the above categories takes place. Someone with a mature faith will display an ability to utilize their specific understanding of God, enabling them to react constructively and positively in order to cope meaningfully in times of illness and suffering. Health is also concurrent with the person's level of insights on how the emotional processes and painful experiences affects one's concept of God. In instances where God is perceived as far away, it is because the patient's emotional and physical pain "places" God at a distance, uninvolved, apathetic, and disinterested—the task of pastoral care is to give the assurance of God's closeness, love, and care and, more importantly, His involvement and presence, especially in times of illness.

Spiritual health therefore means an empowerment of God, where God Himself is the One who empowers people with a living hope and faith in Him. Hope brings the reality of God in us, the hope of all glory closer—a reality of inhabitational presence of the living God, the body being the temple in which Holy Spirit lives. This theory is fundamental to the Christian theological understanding of spiritual healing as the manifestation of a pneumatological event and reason for a celebration of the power of God manifested through the ministry of His servants.

4.10 Spirituality and Spiritual Healing

How are spirituality and spiritual healing important to Home-Based Care to PLWHA?

This research is undertaken from the presupposition based on the Bible as the Word of God and that our spirituality refers to our connectedness with God, our Creator, and our understanding of His involvement in the human experience. A mature spirituality therefore refers to faith in action, and how we react in our spirit in times of illness and suffering—spirituality focuses in the individual's life as being devoted to God and how they view healing. The Eusebian theory and theological meaning of a Christian spirituality implies:[255]

- Spirituality, as godliness, denotes an existential knowledge of God—knowledge based on obedience to God, where faith is not an abstraction from life, but is displayed in our manner of conduct.
- Spirituality has an eschatological dimension—it functions between a tension of salvific truth and daily life, a "struggle" which reflects the character of the development of faith with spirituality relating to both justification and the sanctification of our faith.
- Spirituality denotes a changed life-style (new ethos)—linked to the ethical dimension of Christian faith that has implications for daily life in relation to fellow human beings.
- Spirituality as piety, is not merely a psychic event of emotional experience—it involves subjectivity and has implications for existential and human dimensions of Christian faith—spirituality is therefore the expression of a living faith, which is fulfilled *Coram Deo* (in the

---

[255] Louw (2009), 56.

presence of God) and is expressed and experienced in the fellowship of believers.

This research strongly recommends a Christian spiritual healing paradigm in Home-Based Care that focuses on spiritual healing of life centered around the theological perspectives of:

1. Spiritual healing as a new state of being based on the fact that if anyone is in Christ he/she is a new being (2 Cor. 5:17).
2. Spiritual healing as a new state of mind with *Shalom* being the contentedness with God and life: "for He Himself is our peace" (Eph. 2:14, NKJV).
3. Spiritual healing as a new attitude and way of living producing the fruit of the Spirit— "love, joy, peace, patience, kindness, goodness, faithfulness, gentleness, self-control" (Gal. 5:16; 22–23, NKJV).
4. Spiritual healing as wholeness, purposefulness and direction— "For in this hope we were saved" (Rom. 8:24, NIV).

In a successful Home-Based Care program, Christian spiritual healing with its dimensions of peace (*shalom*), healing (*habitus*), and wholeness (*telos*, meaning) should therefore emanate from the paradigm of existential, life dimensions of healing. Prof. Louw's model of an existential approach to healing is therefore the proposed model for a contextual pastoral care and counselling approach in a ministry to PLWHA for the Seventh-day Adventist Church in South Africa.

Having discussed the role of coping with poverty, illness, crisis, and suffering as an art, and having provided examples of God-images as structures for conceptions of God, and having provided a presupposition of Christian spirituality based on the Scriptures as the Word of God, namely the Bible, we will look at *Cura Vitae* as cure of soul in life care, as an essential and effective tool in pastoral ministry and care in the contextual Home-Based Care to PLWHA.

4.11 An Existential Approach: *Cura Vitae*—Life Dimensions of Healing

A further reflection for a theological consideration in Christian spiritual healing would take into account the impact of *existential issues* of life:

4.11.1 Existential Dimensions of Life

- When the existential threat of *anxiety* as the fear of being rejected is present in the dynamics of human relationships—then the basic existential need is *intimacy*: the need to be accepted unconditionally for who you are without the fear of rejection. *Grace* refers to the theology of unconditional love as a healing dimension.[256]
- The existential threat of *guilt* and *feelings of guilt/shame* from our past can potentially destroy our identity and self-esteem. The basic existential need here is *freedom* and *deliverance*. Spiritual healing means *forgiveness* and *reconciliation*.[257]
- *Despair* and *doubt*: a sense of meaninglessness and being robbed of hope—the basic existential need is *anticipation/meaning/expectation*. Spiritual healing offers renewed trust in the faithfulness of God.[258]
- The existential threat of *helplessness* and *vulnerability* refers to helplessness due to being emotionally displaced—the basic existential being need is a *support system*. Spiritual healing offers *koinonia* (fellowship) as therapy.[259]
- Existential threats of *disillusionment, frustration and anger*— the basic existential need is *life fulfilment*. Spiritual healing offers *gratitude(euchatistia)*[260] and *joy* as therapy. In the participation and the celebration of holy communion all threats of anxiety, guilt, doubt

---

[256] 1 Cor. 15:10.
[257] Col. 2:13–14; 2 Cor. 5:18.
[258] Rom. 15:13.
[259] 1 Cor. 12:26.
[260] Holy Communion.

and despair are removed and spiritual healing and forgiveness is celebrated in *koinonia* fellowship with the family of God.

This is illustrated in *Figure 4: Cura Vitae: Christian Spiritual Care: The Pastoral Response to Existential Threats.*

The goal of pastoral care and counselling as gospel ministry is to care for the soul and to bring spiritual healing to suffering humanity. "The sufferings of every human being are the sufferings of God's child, and those who reach out no helping hand to their perishing fellow human beings provoke His righteous anger."[261] In times of illness, disease, and suffering existential threats operate as viruses of the human soul as shown in *Figure 3* (below). PLWHA are confronted with the quest for meaning in life, meaning in illness, and their future destiny. When our basic life needs/being needs are satisfied, we have the courage "to be." This is the resurrection hope which offers the sick sinner new meaning and direction, new goals and reason to have joy and gratitude.

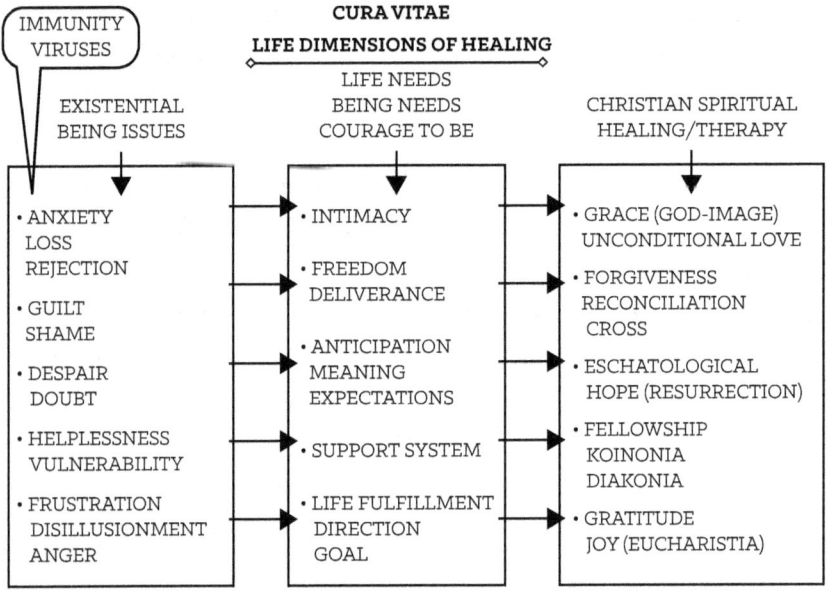

Figure 3: *Cura Vitae*: Cure of Soul as Life Dimensions

---

[261] White, *The Desire of Ages*, 825.

A Christian spirituality based on the existential approach aims to remove anxiety, guilt, and shame, helplessness and vulnerability, frustration, disillusionment, and anger, providing believers life fulfilment and leading individuals saved from death and despair into an attitude of gratitude with the joy and assurance of acceptance into the family of God through *koinonia* fellowship.

4.11.2 Schematic Summary: *Cura Vitae*—Life Dimensions of Healing

Five Viruses of the Soul that endanger spiritual health:

1. *Anxiety*: brings the fear of isolation and loneliness.
2. *Guilt* and *guilt feeling and shame*: rendering a low sense of self-worth.
3. *Despair* and *doubt*: the experience of meaninglessness.
4. *Helplessness* and *vulnerability*: the experience of depression.
5. *Frustration, disillusionment*, and *anger*: experiences of unfulfilled needs causing disappointment.

In *Figure 4* (below), Prof. Louw's *Cura Vitae* model of *life dimensions of healing* clearly indicates the Christian spiritual, pastoral response as intervention in the human predicament—where the soul destroying immunity viruses cause life-threatening being needs, pastoral care effectively satisfies the soul's need of intimacy, freedom, and deliverance, giving the suffering one new meaning, anticipation, life fulfilment, and new direction—therefore *koinonia* fellowship and *diakonia* not only becomes a space where the worship of God takes place but also a space of grace and healing where victory over sin, *Cura Vitae* is celebrated at the joyful Holy Communion instituted by Christ Himself in gratitude and with eschatological hope.

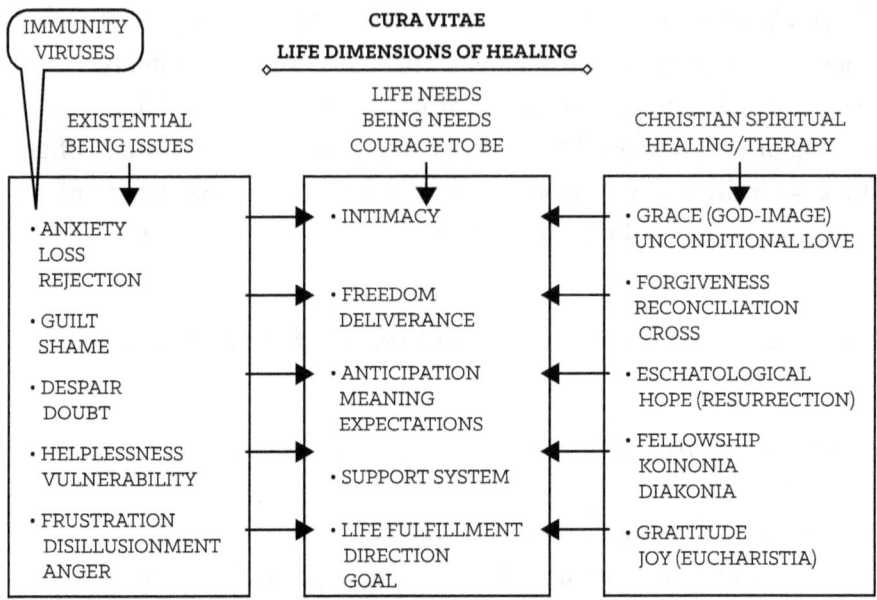

Figure 4: *Cura Vitae*: Christian Spiritual Care and healing as the Pastoral Response to Existential Threats

The power of love is seen in all occasions of Christ's healing, and only by partaking of that love, through faith, can we become instruments of His work and impart the same grace which Christ bestows on us, to others in pastoral care. If we neglect to link ourselves in divine connection with Christ, the current of life-giving energy cannot flow in rich streams from us to the people. In instances where the church might have failed in its mission or overlooked, ignored or neglected the sacred duty of caring for the sick both in the church and the community, Ellen G. White encourages the church to "take His yoke is one of the first conditions of receiving power. The very life of the church depends on its faithfulness in fulfilling the Lord's commission. To neglect this work is to surely invite spiritual feebleness and decay. Where there is no active labor for others, love wanes, and faith grows dim."[262] This serious statement is a timely wake-up call for the church to engage in active ministries reaching the feeble and

---

[262] White, *The Desire of Ages*, 824, 825.

the infirmed in our communities as we rely on the promises of God to be with even till the ends of the earth.

4.11.3 Promissio Therapy

"*Promissio*" therapy has as its root word promise and refers to the healing dimension of God being true to His promises as revealed in His Word, guaranteed by His faithfulness and accompanied by the affirmation of the covenantal events throughout Scripture, such as baptism and the holy communion. It is expressed in the lives and actions of His children when it comes to ethical issues of justice and reconciliation, as well as living according to the fruit of the Spirit. As we lay hold and grasp these promises of God our faith in them will be exemplified and displayed in attitude, behavior and the transformation of our actions. "*Promissio*" therapy operates from within our being functions and activates an intense courage to be.[263]

> Through the goodness and mercy of Christ the sinner is to be restored to the divine favor. God in Christ is daily beseeching men to be reconciled to God. With outstretched arms He is ready to receive and welcome not only the sinner but the prodigal. His dying love, manifested on Calvary, is the sinner's assurance of acceptance, peace, and love. Teach these things in the simplest form, that the sin-darkened soul may see the light shining from the cross of Calvary.[264]

Christian spirituality through *promissio therapy* offers healing to patients. *Cura Vitae* as spiritual therapy brings the helpless, vulnerable individuals into the *koinonia* fellowship and reconciliation with the priesthood of believers. Where grace abounds in actions of unconditional acceptance and love, guilt is removed and forgiveness offers freedom and reconciliation. Despair and doubt turns into glorious eschatological hope.

---

[263] https://1ref.us/sv (accessed 5/6/2019).
[264] White, *Selected Messages, Vol. 1*, 178.4.

How can we convert the theory of *Cura Vitae*, healing of life and the concepts of God-images into a relevant compassionate Home-Based Care ministry of PLWHA and those affected by the HIV and AIDS epidemic in South Africa? I am of the opinion that these useful tools discussed in Chapter four are vital components in Home-Based Care. I suggest that the Seventh-day Adventist Church in South Africa gives consideration to the adoption of Prof Louw's theological reframing of power: *Cura Vitae* as a way forward and new ecclesial approach to contextual Home-Based Care to PLWHA in South Africa. This would relieve the burden carried by district pastors while enhancing pastoral care to those in need of care.

4.12 Home-Based Care Programs in the Seventh-day Adventist Church: An Answer to the Challenge of HIV and AIDS in South Africa

In Chapter one the statement of the problem of "How can the Seventh-day Adventist Church engage the community of faith in pastoral care to those who are living with HIV and AIDS and how can the church initiate a communal contextual Home-Based Care to cater for PLWHA?" has been presented.

1. The core objective of the formulation of a contextual Home-Based Care programme within the Seventh-day Adventist Church in South Africa has been stated under heading 1.10 Objectives of this research.
2. Secondly the aim was to show how that the capacity concepts of Health and a Ministry of Healing can be used by the Seventh-day Adventist Church in South Africa to construct a successful contextual Home-Based Care programme. Under heading 1.8 Basic Research Questions, the question was raised: "What are the theological and ecclesiological implications for being the church in poor communities with a lack of care facilities and health facilities?" Under the auspices of their Personal Ministries department all departments for ministry in the Seventh-day Adventist Church should train and engage their

members to care for PLWHA in the comforts of their own homes and to mobilise their resources needed for socio-economic relief and empowerment to the PLWHA and their families. The church's potential to achieve this aim has been highlighted in Chapter Two.

3. Thirdly the aim was to show how the Seventh-day Adventist Church can interculturate her pastoral strategies so as to respond effectively to the challenges posed by the HIV and AIDS epidemic in South Africa. Chapter two has indicated that in spite of prior challenges the segregated church faced during an apartheid era, the Seventh-day Adventist Church in South Africa has succeeded in a long struggle towards being a united and merged church in 2005. I believe that the decades of merger talks distracted the church from its focus on mission and has greatly retarded their effectiveness and involvement in ministries to PLWHA in South Africa. Meanwhile thousands have died and the rapidly spreading epidemic of HIV and AIDS made South Africa the epicentre in the world. Like other denominations the Seventh-day Adventist Church has PLWHA among her own members in need Home-Based Care and of pastoral care. However, having discussed the important pillars of Adventism and highlighting the mission of the church through various metaphors, the Seventh-day Adventist Church in South Africa should now make drastic efforts to educate, train, empower and engage all her members in HIV and AIDS ministries, and mobilise them via all the existing departments of the local congregations under the umbrella and auspices of their Personal Ministries department.

4. Finally, the aim was to demonstrate how that the Seventh-day Adventist Church in South Africa can mobilise her members in effective ministries to PLWHA, by becoming volunteers in the contextual Home-Based Care programme. The Seventh-day Adventist Church claims to be the *Church of the Living God*[265] on earth upholding doctrines based

---

[265] Rev. 14:12: "Here is the patience of the saints: here *are* they that keep the commandments of God, and the faith of Jesus."

Sola Scriptura, i.e., the Bible and the Bible alone as an only creed,[266] and having *"The Gift of Prophecy:*[267] One of the gifts of the Holy Spirit is prophecy. This gift is an identifying mark of the remnant church and was manifested in the ministry of Ellen. G. White. As the Lord's messenger, her writings are a continuing and authoritative source of truth which provide for the church comfort, guidance, instruction, and correction. They also make clear that the Bible is the authority and standard by which all teaching for spiritual life and experience must be tested."[268] Therefore should the Seventh-day Adventists follow these Twenty-Eight Fundamental Beliefs as doctrine and practice, then every believer a minister means that every believer will become a volunteer according to Christ's great commission. This means that every church member must be encouraged to have an active part and volunteer in gospel ministry, which includes caring for the sick of our communities in their home and caring for their needs – and this is a ministry which includes PLWHA and their families.

This means that the church should educate, train and empower its members adequately for the all-encompassing challenges posed by the HIV and AIDS epidemic. I have examined how other existing ecclesiologies successfully operate Home-Based Care programs and am confident that the Seventh-day Adventist Church should utilize its resources in combined efforts along with other existing ecclesiologies to stem the tide of the HIV and AIDS epidemic and thereby act in accordance with the ultimate call of God—mediating God's kingdom on earth through caring ministries and intervention programs.

Through this research it was interesting to examine the interplay between Seventh-day Adventist spirituality and African spirituality, and

---

[266] Fundamental Belief No. 1, https://1ref.us/sw (accessed 5/6/2019).

[267] Rev 19:10: At this I fell at his feet to worship him. But he said to me, "Don't do that! I am a fellow servant with you and with your brothers and sisters who hold to the testimony of Jesus. Worship God! For it is the Spirit of prophecy who bears testimony to Jesus." See Fundamental Belief No. 18.

[268] https://1ref.us/sw (accessed 5/6/2019).

how both these can help us understand health and healing in the context of the HIV and AIDS epidemic in South Africa, thus engaging the church more actively in successful ministries to PLWHA.

1. This final chapter has expounded extensively on the mandate of the Scriptures as the primary and pivotal calling of the church to engage in the medical missionary work to PLWHA. Pastoral care strategies in multicultural has been adequately discussed as essential for contextual ministries to the people of South Africa. The importance of sensitivity to and education in African spirituality has been addressed and various theories of Professor Daniël Louw, of *A Pastoral Hermeneutics of Care and Encounter, A Theological Design for Basic Theory, Anthropology, Method and Therapy and Cura Vitae,* presented as power tools in pastoral care should be of great help to the Seventh-day Adventist Church in South Africa in the formulation of a successful Home-Based Care ministry as a new ecclesial direction to an HIV and AIDS ministry have been cited.

2. The ultimate aim of this research therefore remains that the Seventh-day Adventist Church in South Africa should give immediate attention to the urgent call of, *"Mi-Yittan,"* OH, If only my people will hear the voice of God calling us as a church to respond to the desperate need of humanity in crisis: PLWHA in need of the healing touch of *Yahweh Rophe*—our Lord Jesus who gave His life for us all – and through our ministries of compassion in Home-Based Care bring Immanuel, God with us to PLWHA and their families. God has blessed and equipped the Seventh-day Adventist Church with sound doctrines of health and healing based on the Scripture and the Spirit of Prophecy as a means to an end and as a lesser light leading us to the greater light, the Scriptures:

> The Seventh-day Adventist Church views "church" as the community of believers who confess Jesus Christ as Lord and Saviour. In continuity with the people of God in Old

> Testament times, we are called out from the world; and we join together for worship, for fellowship, for instruction in the Word, for the celebration of the Lord's Supper, for service to all mankind, and for the worldwide proclamation of the gospel. — Fundamental Belief #12[269]

The world indeed needs today what it needed just over two thousand years ago—a renewed revelation of Christ, and a people willing to do that. Christ came to earth to bring healing, life and light to the world stooped in darkness and to reveal the Father's glory. When the church of God on earth would be willing to follow in the Saviour's steps, to mingle with people as ones desiring their good, showing sympathy for them and to minister to their need "Christ's method alone will give true success in reaching people"[270] and God's will for suffering humanity, will be done on earth.

> Heavenly intelligences are waiting to co-operate with human instrumentalities, that they may reveal to the world what human beings may become, and what, through union with the Divine, may be accomplished for the saving of souls that are ready to perish. — There is no limit to the usefulness of one[s] who, putting self aside, makes room for the working of the Holy Spirit upon his[her] heart and lives a life wholly consecrated to God.[271]

The mission statement of the AAIM ministries discussed earlier in this book in essence sums up the focus and objective of this book: an urgent call to the Seventh-day Adventist Church in South Africa to coordinate, mobilize and engage all its departments, institutions and members in effective caring ministries to PLWHA through Home-Based Care.

---

[269] https://1ref.us/sw (accessed 5/6/2019).
[270] White, *The Ministry of Healing*, 143.
[271] White, *The Ministry of Healing*, 159.

May God grant that *we* become truly consecrated to God in service for humanity. Ultimately, to this end we were called, so that God's eschatological *End* may come.

Maranatha!

4.13 Research Findings

1. This research revealed that the Seventh-day Adventist Church in South Africa has among its members people who are living with HIV and AIDS, and therefore in need of pastoral care and counselling.[272] The research has also clearly revealed that in the broader community, especially poor communities many PLWHA are in need of care.
2. The research also revealed that the worldwide Seventh-day Adventist Church operates on a hierarchical and clerical model (see Figure 1: Organizational Structure of the Seventh-day Adventist Church, page 77) which, particularly in South Africa, becomes a challenge in an effective ministry to PLWHA in local poorer communities, both within and outside of the SDA Church in desperate need of spiritual care, counselling and help. The SDA Church therefore needs to revisit, rethink and restructure itself so as to engage in a model which opts for a less pastor-dependent congregational or grassroots level approach to a successful, contextual Home-Based Care particularly to PLWHA in poor communities. This implies a fundamental shift in the ecclesiological practices of the Seventh-day Adventist Church and an answer to the critical question posed under heading 1.8 Basic Research Questions. This shift would realign the SDA Church with its stated fundamental theology of ecclesiology, calling all members to ministry.

---

[272] Constitution of the South Africa Union (SAU) Association of Adventist People Living with HIV/AIDS (AAPLHA).

3. Also, the Seventh-day Adventist Church has good HIV and AIDS policies in place on administrative levels.[273] These policies, however, are rendered useless unless they are communicated and shared with the congregations and members at a grassroots level—implementation and the success of these policies and strategies will only take place once members are informed, trained, equipped and empowered to engage in compassionate ministries to PLWHA and their families.

4. Furthermore, in order for the Seventh-day Adventist Church in South Africa to successfully and effectively care for its members as well as all other PLWHA in her communities, and more especially those in the poorer communities, the recently merged Church should give study to training its members to engage in cross-cultural situations, and to guard against issues like stigmatization, racism, prejudices and language barriers.

5. This research revealed that with a membership in South Africa of 160,153 members belonging to 1,207 congregations,[274] the Seventh-day Adventist Church has adequate human resources to train and empower in preparation for successful Home-Based Care programs and projects. Also, it has a vast number of professionally skilled people in their congregations who can assist with the training of its members in pastoral care, counselling, and volunteer work in a contextual HBC program. With these resources available, the SDA Church in South Africa needs to shift its ecclesiological focus away from its reorganizational challenges to the equipping, training, and empowering of its membership for ministry.

6. Finally, I have done extensive research and networking with Faith Based Organizations, clinics and facilities of care, have personally worked as pastoral counsellor in several institutions and have, as such, established good relationships and reputation with them. The Seventh-day Adventist Church in their attempts to formulate their

---

[273] https://1ref.us/t4 (accessed 5/6/2019); Constitution of SAU-AAPLHA; HIV/AIDS Ministries, Southern African Union, "Working Policy on HIV/AIDS.".

[274] See Appendix 1.

own HBC programs and initiatives, will do well in seeking the help and expertise of other denominations and FBO's who are currently running successful HBC programs (see the examples under headings 3.3 The JL Zwane Memorial Church, Gugulethu, Cape Town, Responds to HIV and AIDS; 3.4 An Afro-Christian Ministry to People Living with HIV and AIDS in South Africa; and 3.5 The Catholic Church in Rural South Africa and HIV and AIDS).

4.14 Recommendations

Inasmuch as one of the biggest challenges in an HIV and AIDS ministry is to create sustainable models for pastoral care, and to adequately equip pastors, caregivers, and stakeholders with skill to effectively minister to PLWHA, this research proposes that the Seventh-day Adventist Church in South Africa has the distinguishing potential to develop a successful Home-Based Care program and to mobilize her members in such a ministry.

Magezi and Van Dyk propose the following three different models of Home-Based Care:[275]

- *The integrated Home-Based Care model* is an approach which links all the service providers with PLWHA and their families in a continuum of care. In this model the patient and family are supported by a network of services, i.e., community caregivers, clinics, hospitals, support groups, NGOs, CBOs, and FBOs as well as by the larger community. This integrated approach allows for referral between all partners and helps to build trust. It also ensures that community caregivers are trained, supported, and supervised.
- In the *single-service Home-Based Care model* there is one service provider, usually a clinic, hospital, NGO, FBO, or church, that provides HBC by recruiting and training volunteers and brings them in

---

[275] Magezi (2005), 219, and Van Dyk (2008), 334, 335.

contact with the PLWHA at home. Many HBC programs start this way and build their way up to offer integrated care as they recruit other partners.
- *Informal Home-Based Care setting* refers to an approach where families care for their loved ones at home, with informal assistance from their network. Nobody has any specific training or external support and there is no formal organization or supervision of the care. Informal care can be difficult because the primary caregiver often lacks the necessary knowledge, skills, and emotional support needed to care for PLWHA.

As much as Van Dyk points out *the integrated model* as the ideal approach for quality physical care and psychological support for PLWHA, I would suggest that the Seventh-day Adventist Church start with the single-service Home-Based Care model while they seek to recruit other partners, and thereby develop a more integrated HBC program. The reason for opting to start with the *single-service HBC model* is that it enables the local church to begin on a small scale that is easier to implement successfully, and to thus provide a solid foundation for possible later development. It is important that the local church establishes a need by doing a local needs assessment survey. The current policies of the General Conference on HIV and AIDS cannot all be implemented by a given church on the local level. The South African situation is unique, being the epicenter of the HIV and AIDS epidemic. Therefore, they have to structure their Home-Based Care programs to meet the local needs of PLWHA. Establishing good working relationships with hospitals, clinics, churches, NGOs, FBOs, and any other potential organization, is helpful in working towards an *integrated service model*. As the local *single-service HBC project* grows and develops in partnership with other local service providers, it can be restructured according to the local needs into the *integrated model*.

Arising from this research study the following recommendations and suggestions are offered:

1. That the Seventh-day Adventist Church in South Africa will acknowledge that their active involvement in ministries to PLWHA is a social responsibility and moral obligation. The advocacy here is that, in line with their mission and calling, every congregation, especially those in poor communities, should formulate an HIV and AIDS ministry and participate in Home-Based Care programs providing pastoral care to PLWHA in their congregations and in local and neighboring communities.
2. That the Seventh-day Adventist Church embraces a ministry to PLWHA and urgently invests in training programs for pastors, lay counsellors, caregivers, and volunteers in Home-Based Care, healthcare, and spiritual guardianship. Knowledge is power and the empowerment of church members in ministries to PLWHA and their families as well as other terminally ill patients will lighten the burden of pastors in large districts. The advocacy here is for members training as missionary volunteers and recruited for Home-Based Care—the Seventh-day Adventist Church should involve all their departments and enlist members for caring ministries.
3. That the merged Seventh-day Adventist Church in South Africa find ways to celebrate their diversity and enhance cross-cultural ministries. I advocate for the training of leaders and members in intercultural communication skills as a means to break down existing language barriers, prejudices, and attitudes that might hamper effective compassionate ministries to PLWHA and all others in need of pastoral care. The advocacy here is for an empowered and unified task force in the service of God in South Africa.

4. That the SAU and local conferences of the Seventh-day Adventist Church take responsibility for the establishment of regional, district, and local HIV and AIDS offices and centers. The General Conference, AAIM, SAU, and AAPLHA have excellent HIV and AIDS policies in place, which the church should communicate to all its members at a grassroots level and implement. Also, to encourage local churches to become centers of hope and influence in their communities, offering care to PLWHA and their families affected. The advocacy here is for localized HIV and AIDS centers of hope and healing.
5. That the pastors and leaders of the Seventh-day Adventist Church in South Africa befriend and partner with the pastors and leaders of other existing faith communities and join hands in ministries to PLWHA and stem the tide of a fast-spreading HIV and AIDS epidemic through AIDS-prevention campaigns and awareness projects in their communities. The advocacy here is for unified strategies to fight the spread of HIV and AIDS.
6. That the Seventh-day Adventist Church opens its doors on weekdays, offering counselling services, health and lifestyle training, Bible studies, and spiritual support to PLWHA and their families as well as members of the extended community. The advocacy here is for a Seventh-day Adventist church to operate as a multipurpose center and/or Faith Based Organization that is open during weekdays for the community.
7. That the pastors and leaders of the Seventh-day Adventist Church in South Africa study the worthy theories in pastoral care by Professor Daniël Louw, presented in this research study as power tools in the theological reframing of power in pastoral ministry, not only to PLWHA but in all other areas of practical theology, pastoral counselling, and care. The advocacy here is for the training of pastors and leaders as skilled professionals in pastoral care and counselling.

4.15 Further Study

1. The viability and feasibility of local Seventh-day Adventist churches in poor communities operating as multipurpose Faith-Based Organizations and centers of influence, offering health care and social services on weekdays to their local communities in South Africa.
2. Further research studies on the relevance and validity of the writings and teachings of Ellen G. White on health, healthful lifestyle, and health-care in the twenty-first century.

4.16 Conclusion

Despite the continued advances in the fields of science, medicine, and associated professional health care services, the challenges of human diseases in epidemic proportions, more specifically HIV and AIDS, still present us with a need to care for persons, families, and communities afflicted with illnesses. An urgent need exists to respond to the quest for meaning in human suffering and the restoration of human dignity before God in our approaches to ministry and therapy across the cultural divides.

The Christian pastoral counsellors and caregivers have the Scriptures as our primary frame of reference providing us with Biblical historical accounts of *YHWH Rophe* as the Great Physician, Perfect Counsellor and Perfect Role Model: Jesus Christ our Lord.

The culture of the gospel is one that sees the former barriers of racial divides and African cultural differences or indifferences as opportunities for spiritual healing, growth, and transcendence in setting us free, and moving the Seventh-day Adventist Church in South Africa towards truly being and becoming *koinonia* to PLWHA: a place where God's grace lives. The church of God on earth in every aspect and manner of being is the place where *agape love*, unconditional acceptance, healing and forgiveness, spiritual encounter, reconciliation, worship of God the Creator, and eschatological hope of the advent of Christ's coming bring us all, sinners and saints alike, into the priesthood of believers and into unity of Community in Christ.

In Christ we are all one ... Father make us one!

Appendices

APPENDIX 1

Organizational Structure of the Seventh-day Adventist Church

*SAU Pastoral Statistics Report

REPORT OF THE MINISTERIAL ASSOCIATION PRESENTED TO THE FIFTH BUSINESS SESSION OF THE SOUTHERN AFRICA UNION CONFERENCE

Mr. Chairman and Assembled Delegates,

This report of the Ministerial Association covers the periods of both that of my predecessor, Ps. Eddie Baron, who served up till April 2014, and my tenure.

During 2011 a strategic plan was drawn up that was informed by the GC Ministerial Department mission and objectives and served as the basis for the operations and functions of the department.

The Mission Statement of the Association states that its prime function is "to minister to its Pastors, Pastoral Families, Retired Pastors, and local church Elders." As "the Pastor's Pastor," the Association Secretary works through and with his counterparts at conference level to fulfill the Vision of the Association, which is to "encourage pastors and elders of the flock of God, to motivated, vibrant, committed, and spiritual leadership."

In addition to the Pastors and local church Elders, the GC Ministerial Association, through the GC EXCOM, has also placed the training and

Organizational Structure **195**

support of deacons and deaconesses under the umbrella of the Ministerial Association.

Pastoral Statistics[276]

Table 1: Number of Pastors

Total Number of Pastors	328
Pastors Per Member Ratio	554 (SID – 2,042)
Pastors Per Church Ratio	6 (SID – 14.6)
Members Per Population Ratio	419 (SID – 102)

Table 2: Pastors Retiring Within 10 Years

Pastors of Retirement Age (65+)	21
Pastors to Reach Retirement Age within 5 years	23
Pastors to Reach Retirement Age within 6–10 years	30

Table 3: Employment Patterns for Past 10 Years

Total Number of Pastors Employed Last 5 Years	113
Average Rate of Employment Per Year Last 5 Years	22.6
Total Number of Pastors Employed Last 6–10 Years	54
Total Number of Pastors Employed During Past 10 Years	167
Average Employment Rate Per Year for Past 10 Years	16.7

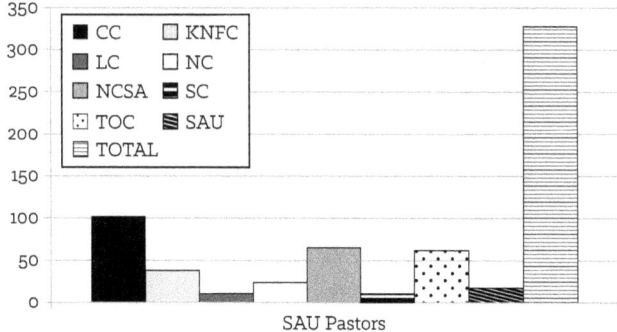

Figure 1: Number of Pastors in SAU

---

[276] Statistics accurate as of 2015.

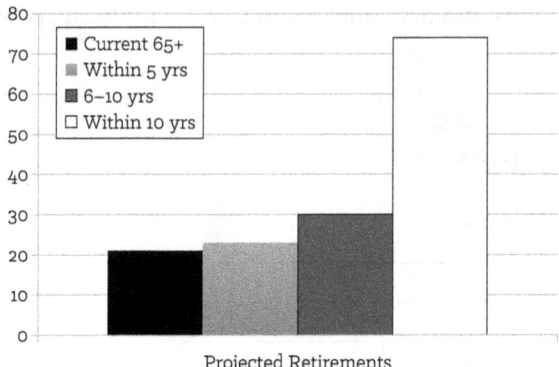

Figure 2: Projected Number of Pastors Reaching Retirement Age up to 2025

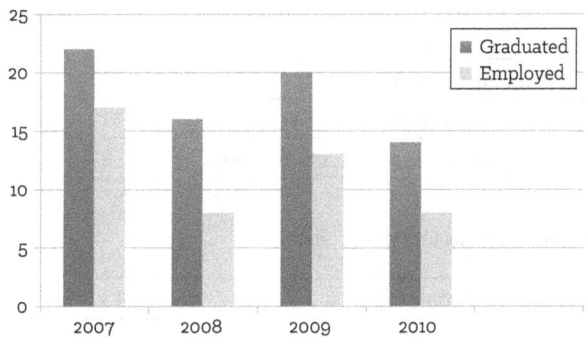

Figure 3: Graduation vs. Employment

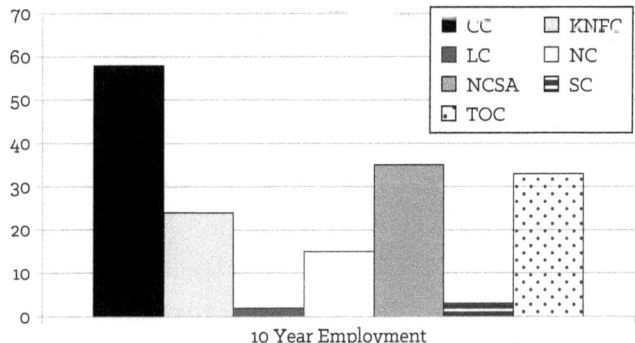

Figure 4: Ten Year Employment Per Conference

Internship

The SAU wishes to see the internship policy being uniformly and consistently applied across all the conferences to ensure that no inexperienced graduate is placed in a district or over a church on his or her own. It is not fair to the graduate or the church. The world Church has a program to allow interns to gain experience, be exposed to working with different seasoned pastors and to be given the opportunity to become involved in the various aspects of ministry under a controlled environment.

New ministerial interns were brought to the SAU offices in Bloemfontein at the beginning of each year during this term for orientation, during which time various speakers dealt with different aspects of their work. In addition, the different conferences conducted internship orientation programs to induct them into the work within the local conference.

Ordinations

Ordination is the church's recognition of the call to full time gospel ministry. During this term the following graph indicates the number of pastors ordained to the ministry:

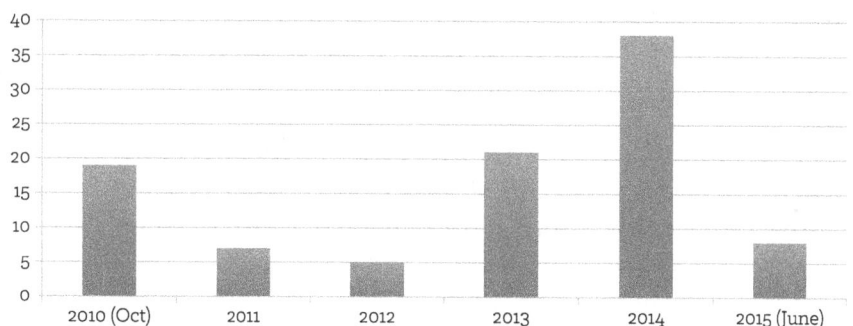

Figure 5: Ordinations Per Year 2010–2015

The total number of pastors ordained over the five-year period was fifty-eight.

In addition to the ordained pastors, who carry ministerial credentials, the ministerial employees are categorized as ministerial interns, licensed pastors, and commissioned ministers' credential.

Withdrawal of Credentials and Resignations

Regretfully we need to report that during this term the ministerial credentials of ten pastors were withdrawn for various reasons.

Ministerial Employees' Meetings and Conventions

Within each conference, ministerial employees' meetings were conducted, which served as vehicles for spiritual refreshment and professional development. In addition, the SAU organized and conducted a Union-wide Ministers and Spouses Convention at Hartenbos in February 2012.

In August 2015 the Association, in conjunction with the president's office, convened a pastoral consultation meeting for all pastors, administrators, and directors. The purpose of this consultation was to review and inform the pastoral corps with regard to the actions and decisions taken at the GC Session held in San Antonio, Texas. The particular areas that were focused on were:

1. The amendments to the Church Manual;
2. Adjustments to the Twenty-eight Fundamental Beliefs;
3. The vote on the action with regard to the ordination of women to the pastoral ministry as it relates to the divisions and its implication for the role of women in leadership within the SAU.

Training Programs and Resources

1. In conjunction with the Health Ministries Department, two **Mental and Emotional Health Training for Pastors Conferences** were held at Bloemfontein featuring national and international speakers.

These conferences focused on sensitizing the pastoral corps on the various mental and emotional health challenges faced by their constituencies. In addition, they alerted the pastors to their own need for mental and emotional health. These conferences were a world first for the SDA church.
2. **Marriage Officers Training.** All marriage officers were brought together to review the legal and ecclesiastical responsibilities and processes to be followed by pastors who are registered as marriage officers.
3. **Elders' Convention.** Following the Convention held in Hartenbos in February, an Elders' Training Convention was held at the same venue with Dr. Jonas Arrais, GC Ministerial Association Associate Secretary responsible for Elders' Training, serving as the main presenter.
4. *Ministry Magazine, Elders' Digest, Shepherdess Journal, Elders' Handbook, Deacon's and Deaconess's Handbook.* The Association is responsible for the management of the subscription of these resources to the different groups under the umbrella of the Ministerial Association.

The *Deacon's and Deaconess's Handbook* is a new publication and seeks to serve as a resource manual for deacons and deaconesses, recognizing the important role and function they play within the church.

Pakia, Shepherdesses, And Retired Pastors

PAKIA

Part of the responsibilities of the Ministerial Association is to promote the association for pastors' kids, called *PAKIA*. This operates within the different conferences at different levels of effectiveness as we strive to recognize the unique needs of this particular group of individuals in the church. The planned PAKIA Convention at union level was cancelled due to the lack of applications and apparent interest in the convention.

The new incoming association secretary, along with the conference ministerial association secretaries, will need to give study to this in order to seek ways of effectively catering for PAKIA.

Shepherdesses

The Shepherdess chapters at the conference levels have organized conferences and retreats, which cater to the particular needs of the spouses of the pastors and administrators. The SAU was able to attend and give support to those to which they were invited.

Some of these seminars and retreats were held in conjunction with the ministerial employees' meetings.

A recent phenomenon, with the employment of female pastors, is the male pastoral spouse. As a result, the Association will have to reconsider the name of the department that caters for the pastors' spouses, as "Shepherdess" does not, etymologically, seem quite appropriate for the males within this group. This issue needs to be escalated to Division and GC level as a result of the reality of female pastors within the Seventh-day Adventist Church.

Retired Pastors

The Ministerial Association seeks to provide support for the retired pastors and their spouses. Special recognition is given to the activities of this group in the Eastern Cape Region who said farewell to one of their strongest leaders and organizers, Ps. G. T Mdliva, during this year.

A number of our retired pastors still give service—some officially and many unofficially. We highly esteem and value the service given by our veterans and their continued support to the program of the church.

A Retirees Convention scheduled for this year was cancelled due to the pressure of work of the Secretary who carries more than one portfolio. It is hoped that the incoming Association Secretary will be able to see this Convention take place early in the new quinquennium.

Appreciation

1. Appreciation is expressed to all the pastors and their spouses, the elders, deacons, and deaconesses, for serving and ministering to God's church. It is through your service that the environment is created and maintained in which men and women accept Jesus as their Saviour, risen Redeemer, and soon-coming Lord; in which they can grow in their faith; in which they are nurtured into discipleship; in which they use their gifts and abilities to spread the gospel of the Three Angels.
2. Appreciation to the Association secretaries and Shepherdess coordinators at conference level for managing the functions and executing the tasks of the Association.
3. Appreciation to Ps. E. Baron and Mrs. E. Baron for their dedicated service as Ministerial Association Secretary and Shepherdess Coordinator for the larger portion of this quinquennium.
4. Appreciation to Mrs. du Preez for her role as the Shepherdess Coordinator during the latter part of this term.

Thanks be to God for His sustaining grace, unquenchable love, and unfathomable mercy.

Maranatha.
Gerald du Preez
Ministerial Association Secretary

Ratio of Pastors to Churches and Members

Cape Conference[277]

Territory: Ascension, St. Helena Island, and Tristan Da Cunha Islands, and the Eastern Cape (including Mount Curry District in KwaZulu Natal Province), Northern Cape, North-Western Cape (except Mafikeng and Vryburg Districts), and Western Cape Provinces in South Africa. Population: 12,436,319.

102 Pastors[i]
461 Churches
40,528 Members

Calculations: Pastor to Church Ratio 1:4.5; Pastor to Member Ratio 1:397.3; Member to Population Ratio 1:306.9.

Kwazulu Natall-Free State Conference[278]

Territory: The South African provinces of KwaZulu Natal, and Free State. Population: 12,442,058.

38 Pastors
160 Churches
17,480 Members

Calculations: Pastor to Church Ratio 1:4.2; Pastor to Member Ratio 1:460; Member to Population Ratio 1:711.8.

---

[277] https://1ref.us/sx (accessed 5/6/2019).
[278] https://1ref.us/sy (accessed 5/6/2019).

Lesotho Conference[279]

Territory: Lesotho. Population: 1,917,000

10 Pastors
40 Churches
7,740 Members

Calculations: Pastor to Church Ratio 1:4; Pastor to Member Ratio 1:774; Member to Population Ratio 1:247.7.

Namibia Conference[280]

Territory: Namibia. Population: 2,348,000

24 Pastors
91 Churches
18,690 Members

Calculations: Pastor to Church Ratio 1:3.8; Pastor to Member Ratio 1:778.75; Member to Population Ratio 1:125.6.

Northern Conference (Formerly Transvaal Conference)[281]

Territory: The South African provinces of Gauteng, Mpumalanga, Limpopo, Northern, and North-West, and the South West Gauteng, and East Rand Regions. Population: 15,207,557.

65 Pastors
129 Churches
19,025 Members

---

[279] https://1ref.us/sz (accessed 5/6/2019).
[280] https://1ref.us/t0 (accessed 5/6/2019).
[281] https://1ref.us/t1 (accessed 5/6/2019).

Calculations: Pastor to Church Ratio 1:1.9; Pastor to Member Ratio 1:292.7; Member to Population Ratio 1:799.3.

Swaziland Conference[282]

Territory: Swaziland. Population: 1,268,000.

10 Pastors
23 Churches
7,173 Members

Calculations: Pastor to Church Ratio 1:2.3; Pastor to Member Ratio 1:717.3; Member to Population Ratio 1:176.8.

Trans-Orange Conference[283]

Territory: The South African provinces of Free State, North-West, Gauteng, Limpopo, Mpumalanga, and the following towns in the Northern Cape Province: Barkly West, Danielskuil, Delportshoop, Douglas, Griquastad, Hartswater, Jankempdorp, Katu, Kimberly, Kudumane, Kuruman, Pampierstad, Postmansburg, Ritchie, Salt Lake, and Warrenton. Population: 13,618,066.

62 Pastors
282 Churches
40,861 Members

Calculations: Pastor to Church Ratio 1:4.5; Pastor to Member Ratio 1:659; Member to Population Ratio 1:333.3.

---

[282] https://1ref.us/t2 (accessed 5/6/2019).
[283] https://1ref.us/t3 (accessed 5/6/2019).

APPENDIX 2

Departments in the Seventh-day Adventist Church for Ministry

Children's Ministries

Children's ministries develop the faith of children from birth through age fourteen, leading them into union with the Church. It seeks to provide multiple ministries that will lead children to Jesus and disciple them in their daily walk with Him. It cooperates with the Sabbath School and other departments to provide religious education to children and fulfills its mission by developing a variety of grace-oriented ministries for children that are inclusive, service-oriented, leadership-building, safe, and evangelistic.

Communication

Communication ministry calls for the support of every layperson, Church employee, and Church institution. The communication department promotes the use of a sound program of public relations and all contemporary communication techniques, sustainable technologies, and media in the promulgation of the gospel.

Education

Church entities operate schools from kindergarten through university levels for the purpose of transmitting to students the Church's ideals, beliefs, attitudes, values, habits, and customs. The source, the means, and the aim of Adventist education are a true knowledge of God, fellowship, and companionship with Him in study and service, and likeness to Him in character development.

Home and School Association—A church with a school shall establish a Home and School Association, the purpose of which is to provide parent education and unite the home, the school, and the church in endeavors to provide Christian education for the children. Parents of students, school patrons, and church members should be encouraged to be active members of the association.

Family Ministries

The objective of family ministries is to strengthen marriage and the family. The family was established by divine creation with marriage at its center. As the primary setting in which values are learned and the capacity for close relationships with God and others is developed, its health is vital to the Church's disciple-making mission.

Family ministries upholds the biblical teaching related to the family and lifts up God's ideals for family living. At the same time, it brings an understanding of the brokenness experienced by individuals and families in a fallen world. The department facilitates understanding, unity, and love at home and in the family of God. It fosters reconciliation between the generations promised in the Elijah message of Malachi 4:5, 6 and extends hope and support to those who have been hurt by abuse, family dysfunction, and broken relationships. Relational growth opportunities are provided through family life education and enrichment. Individuals, married couples, and families are helped to avail themselves of professional counseling when necessary.

Ministry to families in the local church focuses on premarital guidance for couples, marriage strengthening programs, and the education of parents. Ministry to families also gives attention to the special needs of single parents and stepfamilies and provides instruction in family-to-family evangelism.

Health Ministries

The Church believes its responsibility to make Christ known to the world includes a moral obligation to preserve human dignity by promoting optimal levels of physical, mental, and spiritual health.

In addition to ministering to those who are ill, this responsibility extends to the prevention of disease through effective health education and leadership in promoting optimum health, free of tobacco, alcohol, other drugs, and unclean foods. Where possible, members shall be encouraged to follow a primarily vegetarian diet.

Health Ministries or Temperance Society—In some areas a health ministries or temperance society may be established as a separate entity distinct from Church organizations. The conference health ministries director should be involved in establishing such an entity.

Public Affairs and Religious Liberty

The Public Affairs and Religious Liberty (PARL) Department promotes and maintains religious liberty, with particular emphasis upon liberty of conscience. Religious liberty includes the human right to have or adopt the religion of one's choice, to change religious belief according to conscience, to manifest one's religion individually or in community with fellow believers, in worship, observance, practice, witness, and teaching, subject to respect for the equivalent rights of others.

Publishing Ministries

Publishing ministries coordinates and promotes literature evangelism under supervision of the publishing ministries council and the appropriate publishing organization for the territory. It assists other departments in the promotion, sale, and distribution of subscription magazines and other missionary literature. The department works with the pastor and other departments in planning for systematic ways to involve members in publishing ministries.

Sabbath School

The Sabbath School, the primary religious education program of the Church, has four purposes: study of the Scripture, fellowship, community outreach, and world mission emphasis. The General Conference Sabbath School and Personal Ministries Department distributes the Sabbath School Bible study guide for all age levels, provides designs for Sabbath School programming within the context of the various world division cultures, provides resources and training systems for Sabbath School teachers, and promotes world mission Sabbath School offerings.

Personal Ministries

Personal ministries provides resources and trains members to unite their efforts with those of the pastor and officers in soul-winning service. It also has primary responsibility for programs assisting those in need.

Stewardship Ministries

Stewardship ministries encourages members to respond to God's grace by dedicating all they have to Him. Stewardship responsibility involves more than just money. It includes, but is not limited to, the proper care and use of the body, mind, time, abilities, spiritual gifts, relationships, influence, language, the environment, and material possessions. The department assists members in their partnership with God in completing His mission through the proper utilization of all of His gifts and resources.

Women's Ministries

Women's ministries upholds, encourages, and challenges women in their daily walk as disciples of Jesus Christ and as members of His church. Its objectives are to foster spiritual growth and renewal; affirm that women are of immeasurable worth by virtue of their creation and redemption;

equip them for service; offer women's perspectives on church issues; minister to the broad spectrum of women's needs, with regard for multicultural and multiethnic perspectives; cooperate with other departments to facilitate ministry to women and of women; build goodwill among women to encourage mutual support and creative exchange of ideas; mentor and encourage women and create paths for their involvement in the church; and find ways and means to challenge each woman to use her gifts to further global mission.

Youth Ministries

The various youth organizations of the Church should work closely with the youth ministries department of the conference.

Adventist Youth Society (AYS)—The church works for and with its youth through the AYS. Under the AYS leader youth are to work together in development of a strong youth ministry that includes spiritual, mental, and physical development of each individual. Christian social interaction, and an active witnessing program that supports the general soul-winning plans of the church is also of the utmost importance. The goal of AYS should be to involve all youth in activities that will tie them closer to the church and train them for Christian service.

Adventist Youth Features—To help youth grow in their relationship with Jesus Christ, the youth ministries department arranges age-related programming that provides an environment for development of spiritual gifts.

Adventist Junior Youth Society (AJY)—The objectives of AJY are the training of junior youth for Christian leadership and service and the development of members to their fullest potential. In churches with schools the AJY is part of the curriculum and a teacher is AJY leader or sponsor. When the AJY is conducted in the school, each classroom is considered a society, with students in the lower elementary designated as preparatory members. Upper-elementary students are regular members.

Ambassador Club—The Ambassador Club provides a specialized program to meet the needs of youth, ages sixteen through twenty-one. It offers young people in this age group organization and structure, and promotes their active involvement in the church, locally and globally. The club is designed to strengthen the current senior youth/young adult ministry of the Church. It challenges them to experience and share a personal relationship with Christ, helps them develop a lifestyle that fits their belief system and vocational interest, and provides them with a safe venue for wholesome development of lifelong friendships.

Pathfinder Club—The Pathfinder Club provides a church-centered outlet for the spirit of adventure and exploration found in junior youth. This includes carefully tailored activities in outdoor living, nature exploration, crafts, hobbies, or vocations beyond the possibilities in an average AJY. In this setting spiritual emphasis is well received, and the Pathfinder Club has demonstrated its soul-winning influence. In many churches Pathfinder Clubs have replaced the traditional AJY. If there is a school, the Pathfinder Club should supplement the work of the AJY.

Adventurer Club—The Adventurer Club provides home and church programs for parents with six- through nine-year-old children. It is designed to stimulate the children's curiosity and includes age-specific activities that involve both parent and child in recreational activities, simple crafts, appreciation of God's creation, and other activities that are of interest to that age. All is carried out with a spiritual focus, setting the stage for participation in the church as a Pathfinder.

Bibliography

Adventist Aids International Ministries (AAIM). https://1ref.us/s0 (accessed 5/6/2019)

Baker, Delbert W., ed. *Father Make Us One: Celebrating Spiritual Unity in the Midst of Cultural Diversity*. Nampa, ID: Pacific Press Publishing Association, 1995.

Barnett, T., and A. Whiteside. *AIDS in the Twenty-First Century: Disease and Globalization*. New York: Palgrave Macmillan, 2002.

Berinyuu, A. A. *Pastoral Care to the Sick in Africa*. Frankfurt am Main: Peter Lang, 1988.

Bujo, B. *African Christian Morality at the Age of Inculturation*. Nairobi: Paulines Publications, 1998.

Capps, D. *Pastoral Care and Hermeneutics*. Minneapolis: Augsburg Fortress Publishing, 2011.

Centre for Actuarial Research. "The Demographic impact of HIV/AIDS in South Africa-National and Provincial Indicators for 2006." https://1ref.us/t6 (accessed 5/6/2019).

Chitando, E. *Living with Hope: African Churches and HIV/AIDS 1*. Geneva: WCC Publications, 2008.

Church Heritage Manual. General Conference of Seventh-day Adventists, Trans-Africa Division. Malawi: Malamulo Publishing House, no date.

Cochrane, J. W., J. De Gruchy, & R. Petersen, eds. *In Word and Deed: Towards a Practical Theology of Social Transformation: A Framework for Reflection and Training*. Pietermaritzburg: Cluster, 1991.

CSSR Relations. *AIDS and the Church: Report of Visit to Uganda and Tanzania*. Athlone: CSSR, 1994.

DeBose, Edwin R. *The Seventh-day Adventist Tradition: Religious Beliefs and Healthcare Decisions*. 2002. https://1ref.us/s5 (accessed 5/6/2019).

Douglass, Herbert E. *Messenger of the Lord*. Nampa, ID: Pacific Press Publishing Association, 1998.

Dysinger, William. *Heaven's Lifestyle Today*, Silver Spring, MD: The Ministerial Association, General Conference of Seventh-day Adventists, 1997.

Dube, M. "Talitha Cum! A Postcolonial Feminist and HIV/AIDS Reading of Mark 5:21–43," in *Grant Me Justice! HIV/AIDS and Gender Reading of the Bible*. Pietermaritzburg: Cluster Publications, 2004.

General Conference of Seventh-day Adventists. *Seventh-day Adventists Believe*. https://1ref.us/ss (accessed 5/6/2019).

General Conference of Seventh-day Adventists. *Seventh-day Adventist Minister's Handbook*. Silver Spring, MD: The Ministerial Association of GC of SDA, 1997.

Holmes, Arthur. *The Idea of a Christian College*. Grand Rapids, MI: William B. Eerdmans, 1975.

Herek, Gregory M. "Sexual Orientation Differences as Deficits: Science and Stigma in the History of American Psychology," *Perspectives on Psychological Science* 5, no. 6 (December 2010): 693–699, doi: 10.1177/1745691610388770.

Iliffe, John. *The African AIDS Epidemic: A History*. Athens, OH: Ohio University Press, 2006.

Insel, Paul M., and Walton T. Roth. *Core Concepts in Health*, California: Mayfield Publishing Company, 1991.

Johnson S. S. *Hitting Home: How Households Cope with the HIV/AIDS Epidemic*. Henry Kaiser Foundation and Health System Trust, 2006.

Koehler, L., W. Baumgartner, M. E. J. Richardson, & J. J. Stamm. *The Hebrew and Aramaic Lexicon of the Old Testament* (electronic ed., p. 575). Leiden, NY: E. J. Brill, 1999.

Lartey, E. *An Intercultural Approach to Pastoral Care and Counselling.* London: Cassell, 1997.

Lartey, Emmanuel Y. *In Living Color: An Intercultural Approach to Pastoral Care and Counselling.* London: Jessica Kingsley Publishers, 2003.

Lifestyle Intervention Programs. *Be Free Seminars.* Somerset West: printed by Be Free Lifestyle Inc., 2005.

Llaguno, Alex. "Medical Mission Today in the SID." 2007.

Louw, J. D. "Ethics and AIDS in the Development of Prevention Strategy" in Van Niekerk, ed, *AIDS in Context: A South African Perspective.* Cape Town: Lux Verbi, 1991.

Louw, J. D. *Illness As Crisis and Challenge: Guideline for Pastoral Care.* Doornfontein: Orion Publishing Group, 1994.

Louw, J. D. "Pastoral Care for the Person with AIDS in an African Context." *Practical Theology in South Africa* 10, no. 1 (1995).

Louw, J. D. *"Pastoral Care in an African Context: A Systemic Model and Contextual Approach." Missionaria* 25, no. 3 (1997).

Louw, J. D. *A Pastoral Hermeneutics of Care and Encounter: A Theological Design for a Basic Theory, Anthropology, Method and Therapy.* Cape Town: Lux Verbi, 1998.

Louw, J. D. *Meaning in Suffering: A Theological Reflection on the Cross and the Resurrection for Pastoral Care and Counselling.* Wissenschaften: Peter Lang, 2000.

Louw, J. D. *Cura Vitae: Illness and the Healing of Life in Pastoral Care and Counselling: A Guide for Caregivers.* Cape Town: Lux Verbi, 2008.

Magezi, V. *Life Beyond Infection: Home-Based Pastoral Care to People with HIV-Positive Status Within a Context of Poverty.* Stellenbosch University: Unpublished DTh Thesis, 2005.

Manala, M. J. *An Afro-Christian Ministry to People Living with HIV/AIDS in South Africa*, https://1ref.us/so (accessed 5/6/2019).

Martin, Des. *A Faith-Based Response to AIDS in Southern Africa: The Choose to Care Initiative.* Geneva: UNAIDS, 2006. https://1ref.us/t7 (accessed 5/6/2019).

Mbiti, J. S. *African Religions and Philosophy.* London: Heinemann, 1969.

Nicolson, R. *AIDS. A Christian Response*. Pietermaritzburg: Cluster Publications, 1995.

Nieman, David. *The Adventist Lifestyle: Why It Works*. Hagerstown, MD: Review and Herald Publishing Association, 1992.

Njoroge, N. J. "The Missing Voice: African Women Doing Theology." *Journal for Southern Africa*, no. 99 (November 1997).

Noll, G., Rawlyk and D. Bebbington, eds. *Evangelicalism: Comparative Studies of Popular Protestantism in North America, the British Isles, and Beyond 1700–1900*. New York: Oxford, 1994.

Okemwa, P. F. *The Place and Role of Women in the SDA Church in Kenya*. Kenyatta University: Unpublished Master's Thesis, 2003.

Okemwa, P. *Impact of Adventist Schooling on the Status of Women in Kenya: In Quest for Integrity in Africa*. Nairobi: Acton Publishing, 2003.

Page, Robert M. *Stigma*. Psychology Press, 2015.

Philip, E. "Stigma and Silence of the Church." *African Ecclesial Review* (AMECEA) 48, no.1 (2006). Eldoret: GABA Pub.

Pole, H. L. *Christianity in the Academy: Teaching at the Intersection of Faith and Learning*. Michigan: Baker Academic, 2004

Ramphele, M. *Lying Ghost to Rest: Dilemmas of the Transformation in South Africa*. Cape Town: Tefelberg Publishers, 2008.

Ratsara, Paul. President of Southern Africa-Indian Ocean Division (SID) of Seventh-day Adventists in *Adventist Echo* 5, no. 1 (2007).

Robinson, D. E. *The Story of Our Health Message*. Nashville, TN: Southern Publishing Association, 1965.

Rock, Calvin B., ed. *Perspectives, Black Seventh-day Adventists Face the Twenty-first Century*. Hagerstown, MD: Review and Herald Publishing Association, 1996.

Roth, Ariel A. *Origins: Linking Science and Scripture*. Hagerstown, MD: Review and Herald Publishing Association, 1998.

Rowe, Taashi. "South Africa: Grandmothers with HIV, AIDS Find Support in Churches." Seventh-day Adventist Church Inter-American Division. https://1ref.us/t8 (accessed 5/6/2019).

Saayman, Willem and Jacques Kriel. *AIDS: The Leprosy of Our Time? Toward a Christian Response to AIDS in Southern and Central Africa.* Johannesburg: Orion 1992.

Seoka, J. 1997. African Culture and Christian Spirituality in Guma, M. & L. Milton, eds. An African Challenge to the Church in the 21st Century, 1–10. Cape Town: Salty Print, as quoted in Manala, https://1ref.us/so (accessed 5/6/2019).

South African History Online, "A History of HIV/AIDS in South Africa" (March 21, 2011). https://1ref.us/t9 (accessed 5/6/2019).

Swanepoel, L. *The Origin and Early History of the SDA Church in South Africa, 1886–1920.* UNISA: Unpublished Master's Thesis, 1972.

The White Referendum (1983). Fact Sheet 16, https://1ref.us/s2 (accessed 5/6/2019).

Thomas, Adele and Shirley Mabusela. "Foster Care in Soweto, South Africa: Under Assault from a Politically Hostile Environment." *Child Welfare* (1991). https://1ref.us/ta (accessed 5/6/2019).

UNAIDS. "WHO Aids Epidemic Update & Fact Sheet on HIV/Aids in Sub-Saharan Africa." 2006. https://1ref.us/tb (accessed 5/6/2019).

UNAIDS/WHO. "Report on the Global AIDS Epidemic: Annex 2: HIV/AIDS Estimates and Data. 2006.

UNICEF. "Protection for Orphans and Vulnerable Children." https://1ref.us/ry (accessed 5/6/2019).

Van Dyk, A. *HIV/AIDS Care and Counselling: A Multidisciplinary Approach.* Cape Town: Pearson Education South Africa, 2008.

Veith, Walter J. *Diet and Health: Scientific Perspectives.* Stuttgart: Medpharm Scientific Publishers, 1998.

Walsh, John. "'Methodism' and the Origins of English-Speaking Evangelicalism." In *Evangelicalism: Comparative Studies of Popular Protestantism in North America, the British Isles, and Beyond, 1700–1990*, edited by M.A. Noll, D.W. Bebbington, and G.A. Rawlyk. New York: Oxford University Press, 1994.

Walshe, T. *AIDS in the World.* New York: Oxford, 2009.

White, Ellen G. *Counsels on Diets and Foods*. Hagerstown, MD: Review and Herald Publishing Association, 2009.

White, Ellen G. *Counsels on Health*. Nampa, ID: Pacific Press Publishing Association, 2002.

White, Ellen G. *Faith and Works*. Nashville, TN: Southern Publishing Association, 1979.

White, Ellen G. Manuscript 43. "A Talk Presented by Ellen White in the Battle Creek College Library" (April 1, 1901).

White, Ellen G. *The Acts of the Apostles*. Nampa, ID: Pacific Press Publishing Association, 1998.

White, Ellen G. *The Ministry of Healing*. Nampa, ID: Pacific Press Publishing Association, 2003.

White, Ellen G. *The Desire of Ages*. Nampa, ID: Pacific Press Publishing Association, 1998.

White, Ellen G. *The Great Controversy*. Nampa, ID: Pacific Press Publishing Association, 1998.

Whiteside, Alan, and Clem Sunter. *AIDS: The Challenge for Southern Africa*. Cape Town: Human and Rousseau, 2000.

References: Related Publications

Birkenstock, David. "Short History of the Seventh-day Adventist Church in South Africa," May, 2004.

DuBose, Edwin R., ed. Revised by James W. Walters. *The Seventh-day Adventist Tradition: Religious Beliefs and Healthcare Decisions*. Illinois: 2002. https://1ref.us/s5 (accessed 5/6/2019).

Holmes, Arthur. *The Idea of a Christian College*, Michigan: William B. Eerdmans, 1975.

Mathers, Arnet C. *The Shepherd's Psalm 23 (PAV)*, Calais, Maine: 2015, https://1ref.us/su (accessed 5/6/2019).

McMillen, S. I. *None of These Diseases*. New Jersey: Spire Books, 1970.

Pole, Harry Lee. *Christianity in the Academy: Teaching at the Intersection of Faith and Learning*, Michigan: Baker Academic, 2004.

Sire, James. *Discipleship of the Mind*, Illinois: IVP Books, 1990.

Webb, Patricia. *Health Promotion and Patient Education: A Professional's Guide*. London: Chapman & Hall, 1994.

Xapile, N. "The Faith Based Organization Response to HIV/AIDS: A Case study of the JL Zwane Memorial Church in Gugulethu, Cape Town." MPhil (HIV Management), University of Stellenbosch, 2005.

TEACH Services, Inc.
P U B L I S H I N G
www.TEACHServices.com • (800) 367-1844

We invite you to view the complete
selection of titles we publish at:
www.TEACHServices.com

We encourage you to write us
with your thoughts about this,
or any other book we publish at:
info@TEACHServices.com

TEACH Services' titles may be purchased in
bulk quantities for educational, fund-raising,
business, or promotional use.
bulksales@TEACHServices.com

Finally, if you are interested in seeing
your own book in print, please contact us at:
publishing@TEACHServices.com

We are happy to review your manuscript at no charge.

www.ingramcontent.com/pod-product-compliance
Lightning Source LLC
Chambersburg PA
CBHW071607170426
43196CB00033B/2121